The Choice

the true story of
a mother fighting for her life –
and her child

BERNADETTE BOHAN
with Jane Ross-Macdonald

Newleaf

Gill & Macmillan
Hume Avenue, Park West, Dublin 12
with associated companies throughout the world
www.gillmacmillan.ie

First published by *Element*, an imprint of
HarperCollins*Publishers*, 2005

© Bernadette Bohan, 2005, 2011

978 07171 5015 1

Printed by ScandBook AB, Sweden

The paper used in this book comes from the wood pulp
of managed forests. For every tree felled at least one
tree is planted, thereby renewing natural resources.

A CIP catalogue record for this book is available
from the British Library.

5 4 3 2 1

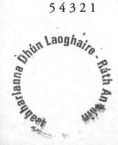

Dedications

To Ger, who is the love of my life

To Richard, Sarah and Julie who are
the meaning of my life

To my little Mammy whose passing away
has left a hole in my life

Note from the publisher

Contents

Acknowledgements   vii
Preface   ix

1	The First Cut	1
2	'It's Just a Big Bruise'	9
3	The Right to Life?	23
4	Loss and Relief	33
5	The Diagnosis	41
6	Steroids: the Good …	49
7	… the Bad …	57
8	… and the Ugly	67
9	New Life	79
10	'A Little Miracle'	91
11	Stress	105
12	Every Woman's Nightmare	119
13	Breaking the News	135
14	'Battle-Stations, Mum!'	151
15	Cruel and Unusual	167
16	Changing Over	189
17	Breaking Through	213
18	Spreading the Word	231
19	Change Simply	251

Resources   281

Acknowledgements

I would like to offer heartfelt thanks to the following people:

Jane Ross-Macdonald for her empathy and dedication which made this book possible.

Wanda Whiteley and Moira Reilly of HarperCollins for their expertise and hard work.

Darragh Hammond for his help and advice from the beginning.

The women – too many to mention by name – who gave unselfishly of their friendship and time when I needed them most.

BERNADETTE BOHAN

Preface

There is nothing special about me. I am an ordinary woman whose life was turned upside down by cancer. I went through the medical treatment like everyone else – steroids, chemotherapy, radiation. Together with my family I went to hell and back. But I recovered, and now feel healthier than I have ever done. Why? Because I took control and made a few simple changes to the way I live my life.

My story starts with a benign breast lump at the age of seventeen. Fifteen years later, with two young children, I was diagnosed with cancer of the lymph system. After I recovered I slipped back into life happy in the belief that I was leading a healthy enough life. I wasn't. And I was told I should never have the third child I so desperately wanted. Years later, after the second, terrible confrontation with cancer I realized I had to do something to help myself and to help my family get through this difficult time. I needed to get back some control, I wanted my husband and children to feel as if they could do something to help too, and I wanted to make each day less painful and help my body all I could. So I read everything I could get my hands on, went to all the talks and lectures I could find, and set about making some real changes.

What happened next amazed me. My arthritis disappeared, I no longer needed my reading glasses, and I was suddenly full of energy. These are small things in comparison with the bigger fight I was having with cancer – but it was a clear indication that the changes I had made were working on my body in a positive way. I realized that if you give your body what it needs it will reward you. I have now been clear of cancer for five years: 'cured' according to the medical profession. I feel healthy, I look well, my eyes are bright, my figure has lost its middle-aged spread, I have more energy than ever before and I am full of vitality.

I was so excited to be feeling this well that wherever I went I told people what I was doing, and how I had helped myself. Gradually people started coming to my house for classes, and I started giving talks. The trickle became a flood, and after I had lectured to capacity audiences at Ireland's largest health show, I appeared on television many times. This stuff was working, people were getting better, and I was receiving hundreds of letters and e-mails testifying to the success of my Change Simply plan each week. I was constantly being asked for a book, a video, an information pack – anything. And eventually I was persuaded to write my story.

So here it is. I think it is an ordinary story, but like all ordinary stories it has its share of heartache and joy, of passion, tenderness and sorrow. I believe every mother will recognize the agonies I went through, and anyone who has confronted illness in themselves or others – particularly cancer – will understand my urgent need to find answers. I have met so many people during the course of teaching the health principles you will read about here that I cannot claim to have had a more tragic life than anyone. I am humbled time and again by the pain of others and by their selflessness in the face of seemingly insurmountable obstacles. I do not feel I deserve the accolades that have been heaped upon me: I am no angel, no guiding light, no healer, although I have been called all of these and more. It just makes me happy to pass on the amazing knowledge I have acquired. I am — and I stress it again — just an ordinary woman who discovered that by making simple choices she could make a difference to herself, and others. I am conscious, though, that the suffering and pain that I went through was, in a sense, a kind of gift.

However, I sometimes think that if I have been given a gift at all, it is the gift of the gab, and indeed I am happiest when I am waxing about these few simple changes that anyone can make. My life is now devoted to telling as many people as I can about the four key steps to a healthier life. Read my story to find out why I had to make the choices I did, and read the health plan to find out how easy it is to change your own life.

The choice is yours.

Chapter One

The First Cut

W hen I was seventeen I discovered a lump in my breast.

This was 1971, and I can't say we were very clued-up on health matters then. Nowadays, of course, just about every woman's magazine has advice and information on breast care, how and when to check for lumps, what to do if you think you have found one, and so on. I shouldn't be surprised if they taught it at school now as well. But back then, this was not the case. Not only were health issues not discussed, they were almost taboo. As a family, we were very self-reliant when it came to sickness. If one of us fell ill or was hurt in some way, my mother would 'doctor' us; there was never any question of going to the doctor.

I remember one summer playing barefoot in the yard outside our house when I felt a sharp stab in one foot. I cried out in pain and limped into the kitchen to tell mum. As I sat down I could see that I was bleeding quite badly. 'You've stepped on a nail!' cried my mother. 'Come here, I'll see to it.' She washed it under the cold tap and reached up in a cupboard for what we kids called her 'Doctor Box'. A few minutes later I was expertly bandaged, and with a kiss from mum I was ready to hobble off to resume my game of hopscotch. I knew I would be all right because she was looking after me: she made me feel totally secure and completely loved. The following day, before I left for school, Mum knelt down beside me. She looked at the wound and changed the dressing. 'Mind you tell them that you went to the doctor,' she cautioned. I nodded. Doctors were expensive, not for the likes of us. Another time I was messing with her sewing machine and managed to plunge the needle right through my finger. Again, Mum sorted it.

When I think about this now I'm astonished that none of us fell prey to tetanus, septicaemia, pneumonia or worse. We led a very rough-and-tumble existence and the boys in particular were often getting hurt. In winter if we caught a chill it was mustard baths and bed, then up again as soon as the colour came back into our cheeks. Perhaps we were lucky, or perhaps today we are all too ready to dash to the GP at the first twinge or sniff.

Whatever, I think it gave us children a strong sense that we were responsible for our own healing, and that getting better happened at home. We were a tight-knit family, and I have very happy memories of those years – my mother doing her best to give us the loving stable childhood she herself had been denied.

I was in the bath when I discovered the lump, quite by chance, in my right breast. I didn't know much, but I had done a bit of reading – in fact I quite enjoyed finding out about anything to do with health – and I knew enough to be concerned. 'Mum, will you have a feel of this?' I yelled out. She came into the bathroom and felt what I was feeling. For once she did not suggest doctoring me herself. 'It's probably nothing, but go get it checked as soon as possible,' she said, frowning. Go to the doctor? Me? This had to be serious.

Thinking back now to my innocent seventeen-year-old self later on that week, lying on the bed in the doctor's surgery trying to take my mind off the examination, I wonder how I would have felt if I had been told then that I would spend hours of my life lying on beds like these. It was so foreign to me to be there in the first place – the smell in the surgery, the doctor cold and matter-of-fact. I was glad that Mum had saved me from this so far. The lurching feeling I felt that day in the pit of my stomach was to come back again and again over the course of my life, and not even Mum could save me from that.

'It's definitely a lump. I recommend we remove it next week.' The doctor's words brought me back to earth. 'It is a fairly simple procedure. You won't feel a thing, and we'll examine the tissue to see what we've got. We need to find out what kind of a lump this is and if we need to do anything about it. Let's see if we can get you booked in for that.'

I walked home that day, my head spinning. It was summer and the golden evening light spread in shafts across the road. I could hear the distant clack of lawn mowers and smell the fresh, herby scent of newly cut grass. A bee buzzed at my head but I walked on, in a daze. This was the first time I had ever faced anything like this, and I knew I was going to have to face it alone. I wasn't a child any more, and this felt like my first test of adulthood.

What was happening to me? How would the operation work? I was so naïve, and I had never had an anaesthetic before. I couldn't imagine how they could take the lump out and not hurt me. Whom could I ask? I thought of my friends, mainly local girls from school. None of them had ever gone through anything like this, and problems like this were not the kind of thing you talked about then. I badly wanted to talk to my big sisters – they would know what was what, but they were married and living a fair step away.

I reached my house and saw my mother leaning over the garden fence talking in hushed tones to a neighbour. She turned and hurried towards me, gathering me up in her arms as I sobbed the news. I was terrified at the prospect of pain, and the idea of having a scar right across my breast for the rest of my life. 'It will be all right, you'll see,' she whispered into my hair. 'I'll never let my baby get hurt. Come on now girl, dry your tears.' I breathed more slowly. How comforting a mother's arms are when things go wrong. Although I thought I was all grown-up, I realized that so much of me was still a child. She would make it better. Nothing bad was going to happen.

A week later I packed a few things carefully into a bag, desperate not to betray my nervousness to my mother who was fussing around me, trying not to show her own fears. 'Have you got everything? What time did they say to be there for? What did they tell you to bring in?' I knew how worried she was but I needed her to be strong for me.

Fortunately the lump was benign. 'It was just a cyst,' explained my doctor. 'These things come up from time to time. Nothing to worry about, but keep checking yourself regularly just in case.'

I suddenly realized that I had been so fixated on the pain and the scar it simply hadn't occurred to me that it might be malignant. I reeled. 'What happens if I get one again?' I managed to ask.

'The only place for a lump in a woman's breast is under the microscope,' he said confidently, as if it was something he had said many times before and would say many times in the future. It was one of those black-and-white statements that I have grown used to hearing from the medical profession.

I think now that perhaps I would disagree with what he said.

After this I checked myself diligently for a year or two, and gradually I found myself doing it only now and then. As I grew older I began to understand how lucky I had been, especially when I heard of others who were not so lucky. The scar faded, and with it my memories of that fearful time.

It was around this time that I met Gerard, the boy who was later to become my husband. I was young, I wanted to have fun, and I wanted to put the whole experience behind me.

Chapter Two

'It's Just a Big Bruise'

Fifteen years later, and my four-year-old daughter Sarah was in a frenzy of excitement. 'Mammy, are we really going on an aeroplane?' she cried. 'Yes, really,' I said, laughing. 'Tomorrow night we'll be up above the clouds.' 'What, up in the sky and all? Will we have beds to go to sleep on? Can I bring all my Barbies?' She rushed up to her room to gather her favourite things. Richard, two years older, was a little more restrained, but I knew from the way he rushed home from his last day at school that he was just as thrilled as she was to be going on their first foreign holiday. Months earlier, back in the dreary Dublin winter, we had pored over brochures searching for somewhere to take the kids to for a fortnight's sun. Usually we went away to friends, or spent holidays travelling around Ireland – but we felt it was time the children had the chance to play on a beach without wearing several layers of clothing or being driven into a coffee shop by drizzle or high winds. So Tenerife it was, and now at last it was July and the school holidays were here.

I had been knocking spots out of the sewing machine for weeks, making up clothes for Sarah. Always full of energy, I had felt particularly well that summer and worked late into the night making sure everything was going to be ready on time. The children's things were laid out carefully on the bed in the spare room: rows of shorts, swimming things, T-shirts and sun hats. Sarah kept peeping in to check that her new sundress with the bright red flowers was still there. 'Will you stop your fiddling and leave those things be?' I kept scolding her. 'Aw, Mammy, I just wanted to see it. Can I try it on again? Pleease?' Her eager face and bright smile always melted my heart. 'Go on then. I've got to go and wash the kitchen floor so you come right down after. Don't mess with my nice neat piles will you now?' I headed downstairs and got on with washing the floor.

I was in the middle of a pre-holiday clean up: I always liked to come back to a pristine house. While I was mopping the floor I pulled the kitchen table towards me rather too quickly and banged the edge of it into my groin, just at the top of my right leg. 'Ouch!' I yelled out, tears stinging my eyes, just as Sarah came running in. 'What is it Mammy, are you hurt?' 'No, it's nothing – just a bash from the table. Now, what are we going to have for dinner?' I rubbed the spot and turned my attention to the potatoes. I thought no more about it until a few days later.

Tenerife could not have been more idyllic. We spent the days relaxing under a huge parasol on the beach next to our hotel, watching the children building great fortresses and dugouts in the sand, or hurtling in and out of the waves. What minor cares we had seemed to melt away in the sun. One morning I looked over to where Ger was lying, marvelling at the way his frown lines had disappeared. He was a good man, a great father. How lucky I was. I breathed a long contented sigh.

'Happy?' he glanced up from his book. 'You bet your life I am,' I answered. 'This is just perfect.' The kids were in heaven – as I watched them capering around I felt so unbelievably content and at peace with the world. We had been married for nine years, and this was just how I dreamed life could be with Ger and the children. At that moment Sarah skipped over to show us a pretty conch shell she had discovered. I examined its pearly interior and held it to my ear, listening for the soft *sshhh* of the sea. 'Listen, Sarah. Can you hear the sea whispering?'

'I can hear it whispering but I don't speak sea language,' she said stoutly, after concentrating for a while with her eyes shut. 'You listen, Daddy.' Ger obliged: 'It's a huge long story,' he said, playing for time. 'Is it a happy story?' she asked. 'No, it's a sad story, but it has a happy ending.' Sarah looked at him expectantly, but any more questions were forgotten suddenly as Richard appeared bearing armfuls of seaweed. The children giggled as they draped the brackish fronds over themselves and waved it at me. 'We're sea monsters, come to drag you away,' growled Richard in his best sea-monster voice. 'Get that slimy stuff away from me!' I cried in mock terror, jumping up. After a momentary scuffle which ended when Ger out-monstered the sea monsters, they wandered off.

Some time later, sitting on the edge of my sunbed, I was watching Richard covering Sarah's legs with sand as she lay in a hollow they had dug. Slowly he sculpted the sandy mound into a mermaid's tail. I did not notice that Ger was staring at my legs.

'What's that, Bernie?' Ger was looking at my groin and frowning. 'What's what?' I asked, shaken from my reverie. He stretched out his hand and touched what was an unmistakable lump on my inner thigh. 'Oh, that. It must be where I got that bump the other day. I was moving the table and bashed myself. It's just a big bruise.' It wasn't bruise-coloured though, and it was very tender to the touch.

'I don't like the look of it,' he said. 'Let's keep an eye on it.' We did – in fact it was hard not to, dressed as I was in swimwear and shorts. Over the next few days it seemed to get bigger and bigger, and was sore if I pressed it. I thought then that it seemed like that only because he had said it. By the end of the holiday it was as big as a golf ball, and almost as hard. Shorts were uncomfortable to wear, and I could feel it chafe when I crossed my legs. I fretted in silence, not wanting Ger or the children to know I was worried. But he could read my mind then – as he still can now – so he knew he had to jolly me along with jokes. 'How's the golf ball this morning? Is it still there? Looks like I'll be collecting on the life insurance money any day now!' Sometimes he even jokingly called it my 'malignant lump'. By making a joke about it he was making it unreal, distancing it from us.

No matter how much I tried to push it to the back of my mind and reclaim the sweet sense of contentment that had overwhelmed me at the beginning of our holiday, I couldn't for the life of me imagine what this lump could be, and a tangible sense of fear started to creep up on me.

On our last day we were having a final drink on the balcony of our hotel room, watching the sunset. We were chatting comfortably about the holiday, and I was enjoying the peace and quiet, knowing the children were both asleep. Ger looked at me. 'I know we've joked about this, but seriously now Bernie, I want you to get that lump checked out as soon as we get home. Make the appointment – let's not mess around here.' He didn't have to tell me – I was as anxious to know what this could be as he was.

Although we had moved house I had not got round to registering with a new doctor, which in hindsight turned out to be a blessing. I drove the few miles back to Ayrefield, where the receptionist gave me an appointment immediately. My doctor was a middle-aged man with kind grey eyes and an old-fashioned reassuring manner. I liked and trusted him: he had always been ready to listen to me and respond to my hunches – something that is hard to find in the medical profession. Years before, when Richard had suffered from eczema, this doctor hadn't foisted kidney-damaging cortisone creams on him, but had allowed me to try to sort it myself through diet. I had read that cutting out dairy products could be beneficial to skin conditions such as eczema, and sure enough Richard's dry red patches disappeared a short while later.

'Hmm,' he said as he examined the lump in my groin. 'This might have been caused by an infection. Have you had a nasty cut at all, on your foot for example?' 'No,' I replied, unable to think of anything. 'Well, you have been abroad and you never know what you might have picked up. I'll put you on antibiotics for a week and I'll see you back here after that, whether or not this lump has gone.' We chatted then for a bit about my holiday and how the children were doing. I rose and thanked him for the prescription. 'Bye now,' I said.

The door clicked behind me, but as I left I heard it open again.

'Mrs Bohan?'

'Yes?' I turned round expectantly.

'Don't not come back,' he warned.

I took the antibiotics and checked the lump daily. That weekend we went to the christening of my sister Aquinas's baby boy, Dean. It was a joyful occasion, and everyone was in high spirits. I didn't mention anything to my mother or sisters of course – there didn't seem any point involving them until I knew what this thing was. At the end of the week it was still there. 'I'm going back to see the doctor,' I told Ger. 'The antibiotics haven't done a thing.'

'Do you want me to come with you? I have a few meetings on today.'

'No, you're all right. I'll be fine. I'll call you when I'm done.'

So I went back to the doctor by myself, trying to ignore a nagging sense of unease.

He felt the lump from all angles, his brow furrowed. 'I think you ought to see a specialist to get this lump properly checked out,' he said. That sounded ominous.

Then I remembered something else. It had almost slipped my mind because of the worry of the lump. 'I've missed a period. Do you think I might be pregnant?'

Ger and I had been toying with the idea of a third child. Sarah was four and it seemed like it could be a good time to start thinking about the next one. It had not been uppermost in our minds, but we had not particularly been trying to avoid having a baby. Because it wasn't a huge deal for us, I hadn't mentioned to Ger that I was late. Yet here I was, suddenly facing the possibility that I may indeed be pregnant. It didn't occur to me that my timing was appalling.

He looked up and I saw a flash of concern cross his face. 'That might complicate things,' he said slowly. 'You'd better come back tomorrow with a urine sample to confirm whether or not you're really pregnant.' There was something in his grave expression, and the fact that he phoned then and there to make an appointment with the specialist that made icy fingers creep around my heart. Something was clearly terribly wrong. I didn't want to leave his surgery before getting more information. I needed to know what I was dealing with. I looked at this kind, straight-talking man.

'Please, doctor,' I said, 'I'm worried now. What do you think this might be? I need a straight answer.' There was a long pause. He shuffled his papers for a moment then looked me in the eye.

What he said then shocked me – I was used to doctors being somewhat secretive and evasive in their habit of drip-feeding information to patients.

'I think it's either lymphoma or Hodgkin's disease.'

The words spun through my mind: I had heard of Hodgkin's and I knew it was rare and bad. I had never heard of lymphoma, but I sure as hell was going to find out about it before I did anything else.

I can't remember driving home that day. I must have gone to the school to pick up Sarah, because I know that later on I left her with a neighbour. Richard came out later. I needed to be alone when I phoned Ger at work.

'Ger,' my voice trembled as I held the phone, 'I have some bad news.' I heard him draw breath as he waited for me to go on. I couldn't say the words. 'Stay there. I'm coming right home,' he said. I knew he had guessed what it was.

An hour later we were standing together in our kitchen, arms locked around each other, silent tears falling. I had just told him what had happened. Ger was confused – 'What else did he say?'

'Nothing. That was it. Lymphoma or Hodgkin's.'

'OK. We need to find out what we've got here,' he said eventually, as he reached for the giant medical reference book I kept on the shelf. Like my mother before me, I tried to deal with family health problems myself. Unlike my mother, though, I always wanted to find out all the facts.

This is what we read: *The lymphatic system is one of the body's defence mechanisms. It filters out organisms that cause disease, produces certain white blood cells and generates antibodies. It is also important for the distribution of fluids and nutrients in the body, because it drains excess fluids and protein so that tissues do not swell up.* So far, so good. *A lymphoma is a painless swelling of the lymph nodes in the neck, underarm or groin.* Mine hurt! I rejoiced – perhaps it wasn't this after all.

Other symptoms may include the following: unexplained fever; night sweats; constant fatigue; unexplained weight loss; itchy skin; reddened patches on the skin. Again, I had not had any of these symptoms, most of which sounded to me like flu. I had been feeling better than I had felt in ages. I had loads of energy. Surely this was all a bad dream. I couldn't be ill, could I? There must be some mistake. We read on: *Lymphoma is a general term for cancers that develop in the lymphatic system. It occurs when cells in the lymphatic system become abnormal. They divide too rapidly and grow without any order or control. Hodgkin's disease is one type of lymphoma. There is only one way to tell the difference, and that is when the cells are looked at under the microscope. Both types of cancers can spread to almost any part of the body, including the liver, bone marrow, and spleen.*

Until this moment the words 'lymphoma' and 'Hodgkin's' had been just that, mere words. Now I realized they were both words for cancer.

The Big C.

It hit me like a slap in the face. Dumbstruck, I stared at Ger.

'There's something else I haven't told you yet,' I said. 'I think I'm pregnant.'

Ger's face lit up for a brief moment before darkening. A mass of contradictory emotions was welling up inside him, but he spoke calmly: 'Well, sure that's great,' he said carefully, 'but the most important thing is for you to be well. How certain are you?'

'Well,' I said slowly, 'I've missed a period, I have a painful, dragging feeling here,' I placed my hands over my lower abdomen, 'and I've got a strange metallic taste in my mouth.' He looked dubious, but these were clear signs for me – I had been pregnant twice before, after all. And my breasts already felt fuller and slightly sore. My mind leapt forward: March. The baby would be born in March. I couldn't help but feel excited.

'Bernie,' he said softly. 'Let's not jump to conclusions on either count. We don't know it is definitely Hodgkin's or lymphoma – GPs don't know everything, and there are lots of symptoms in that book you haven't got. Let's wait for the specialist to tell us exactly what's wrong with you. And anything might happen with the pregnancy.'

He was being too calm, too conciliatory. I was touched, but that scared me almost more than the idea that I was going to be ill.

'Well, I'll find out tomorrow if I'm really pregnant, and on Thursday I'm seeing the specialist.' Put like that I thought it sounded perfectly possible for the two different issues to exist side by side. I wanted to sound confident and in control, as if I was taking all this in my stride. Ger smiled with the confidence he always exuded. 'Look, we're in this together. Whatever happens, I'll be here to look after you and the children.'

I could not sleep that night. My doctor's words kept echoing through my mind: *this might complicate things.* Was I pregnant? What would it mean? What was the lump? Could it really be cancer? I was only thirty-two – surely much too young to be given a death sentence. I lay awake for hours, and eventually slipped into a fitful sleep.

I dreamt of my father, who had died when I was twenty-five. In my dream he was once again lying in his hospital bed, ghost-pale and thin. I tried to hug him but I couldn't, because of the mass of tubes snaking into his arms and neck. I couldn't get close enough to him. Suddenly he was sitting up and my sister Aquinas was in the room too. He said to her, 'You used to be my favourite, but this lassie is my favourite now.' Then I was washing him, and he was ashamed, hunched over on the bed. He looked shrunken, defenceless. I felt like I was the only one who could look after him, and I was saying 'Don't worry, you did this for me, it's OK.' He could barely lift up his head but he managed to whisper, 'And I will again, pet, I will again.'

I woke up, my face wet with tears. Dad had died of lung cancer, and I did not know if I was crying for him or for myself. I loved him dearly, so I did. Reaching over for Ger, I buried my head in his chest and felt comforted by his warmth and strength.

Chapter Three

The Right to Life?

I was right. The pregnancy test was positive, but I hardly allowed myself to dwell on it. My mind was a mass of conflicting emotions: it was lovely to be pregnant, but devastating to be facing a major illness. I did my best to blank out both things and absorb myself for the next two days in Richard and Sarah and their little lives.

It was the night before my appointment with the specialist. I cooked Ger's favourite supper – steak, onions, peas and potatoes – spending more time than usual preparing it. Mundane tasks like chopping vegetables calmed me, and as I smoothed the white linen cloth over the table and laid out the dinner plates and glasses it seemed to me that it was possible to lend some order and certainty to our lives. Sitting there later with Ger, the evening breeze drifting in from the open patio doors, I almost felt that everything was all right with the world. It was so perfect, yet so brittle. I wanted to freeze this moment, stop the hands of the clock, and stay just as we were.

We talked about plans for the following day. Ger said, 'I think you had better pack a bag, just in case.' I was surprised. 'But I'm only going in for an out-patient appointment. Even if I need to be admitted it surely won't be straightaway.'

'It won't hurt to be ready. If you bring the bag home again, so much the better.' Ger was adamant. He always likes to be one step ahead of the game, prepared for every eventuality. This is a wonderful quality and was to be crucial for me in the months and years ahead – during my treatment, when I was stumbling weakly through the days, I always knew that Ger was buoying me up, making me feel secure and looked-after. If I fell I knew he would be there to catch me.

We were lucky enough to have private health cover, and we were being sent to a hospital half an hour's drive away. The journey seemed endless, and I sat quietly while Ger chatted away: I knew he was trying to take my mind off things. *Dear God*, I prayed, *Help me to get through this ordeal.* We arrived at the new, modern hospital building with plenty of time to spare. I was amazed at the plush corridors and shiny chrome and glass interior – it looked like the sort of place no one could be sick in. 'I wouldn't mind spending a few days here myself,' joked Gerard. 'It looks like a hotel.' I looked at the signs we were passing. Renal Department. Ear, Nose and Throat. And I remembered the medical book: *Both types of cancers can spread to almost any part of the body…* This was no hotel.

The specialist, or the oncologist as I learnt to call him, was a distinguished-looking man in his early fifties with pepper-and-salt hair. His eyes were penetrating and I sensed a sharp mind and a quick brain. He shook my hand and smiled at me.

'Good morning, Mrs Bohan. I've read your notes. Why don't you start by telling me when you first noticed this lump?' I told him everything I could remember, Ger chipping in from time to time. Then he examined me.

'We'll need to organize a biopsy. No need to worry, it is a simple procedure in which we take a section of tissue and send it off to the lab for analysis. Wait here for a moment while I ask Claire to check the calendar.'

Ger followed him out, saying hurriedly to me, 'I won't be a moment.' I knew what he was doing. He wanted to buttonhole the oncologist himself, and later he told me what transpired.

'Can you do anything tomorrow?' Ger asked him.

'Tomorrow? Not really. It's Thursday today, and Friday is a bit soon to get things sorted. We don't do biopsies at weekends, so I think the soonest we're looking at is Monday or Tuesday.'

'We have a bag packed. If you can fit her in she's all set.' Ger hates waiting, and always wants to get the job in hand sorted. 'I just want to find out what this thing is and get on with it.'

The oncologist was taken aback. 'You've packed a bag? That's efficient. Now, let's see then.'

While he looked at the schedule Ger wondered how to phrase his next question. He decided the direct approach was best.

'You know my wife is pregnant. Tell me if she can have the treatment or … or will she need an abortion? I need to know what our position is.'

'Mr Bohan, it really is too early to discuss anything like that. Let's take this one day at a time. In a few days we will know what we are facing and what the possible treatment might be. Then we can talk about the pregnancy. What I can say is that if she has what I suspect she has, she cannot wait nine months for treatment. And treatment would damage the foetus. My job now is to make your wife well. Would you mind waiting with her while I make some calls?'

We had had a referendum in Ireland on abortion a few years earlier, as a result of which it was confirmed that the unborn baby's right to life was equal to that of its mother. So for Gerard to raise this question was deeply contentious. However, as happened in my case, doctors must not refuse life-saving treatment to any mother even where it is likely that the treatment may damage the baby.

It was clear the oncologist would not say any more at this point. Later he told me that this was quite common: patients would bombard him with questions, desperately wanting to know everything all at once.

'I can't possibly tell them what is ahead of them when they are just embarking on treatment, or sometimes not even needing treatment at all,' he said to me one day. 'Every patient reacts differently, every tumour is different, and it's not very helpful to tell people they are possibly entering the hardest period of their lives. My way of helping them is to take them through each stage as gently as possible – and, hopefully, eventually to cure them.'

We were lucky that Thursday. The oncologist managed to find a surgeon to do the biopsy the next morning, and before I knew it I was upstairs in the ward. After I had been booked in and the various formalities gone through and we were alone, Ger drew the curtains around my bed. He told me what he had asked the oncologist. I was horrified.

'An abortion? Wh-what in God's name are you talking about?'

It may sound odd, but I hadn't admitted to myself the possibility of terminating the pregnancy. I knew it complicated things, that was all. I simply had not faced up to what that might mean in reality.

'Ger, I am carrying our baby. You know there is no way I can get rid of it. I just can't. I haven't got it in me.' I needed time to get my head together – it was all happening too fast. This was the sort of thing that happened to people in movies, not ordinary people like us. I had a mental image of this tiny baby clinging to me, fighting for its life.

'Jesus, Bernie. You have two healthy kids at home. What are you thinking?' I realized that Ger was naturally concerned for me and our children, and his protective instincts were focussed on keeping the status quo. I knew he was trying to introduce me gently to the prospect of not having this child. But he was a man: how could he possibly understand what it was like to be carrying a baby? It was a precious gift. I was a mother, and I was being given a chance to be a mother again. Nothing was more important.

The next morning I was given the pre-med to make me a bit dozy, but as I was wheeled into the operating theatre where the anaesthetist was waiting there was only one thing on my mind. 'Remember I'm pregnant won't you?' I said to him. 'Make sure you don't do anything to harm the baby.'

'Don't worry, Mrs Bohan. It's only a local anaesthetic.' He spoke calmly and soothingly. Nevertheless, I felt sick with fear and anxiety.

After the biopsy I lay in my bed watching the other people in the ward. In the bed opposite me was a woman in her early forties. One of the nurses told me she had leukaemia. 'Say a prayer for her,' she said. I looked at her – her skin was grey, she had no hair, she could barely set one foot in front of the other. She smiled back, and I went over and asked her how she was feeling. She told me about her family, and how she was hoping to go to Australia to see her youngest son for Christmas.

Ger was in and out of the hospital that day, rushing around for the children, bringing me in things, waiting and waiting for the results. We were hoping to hear something that day. The hospital food was amazing (yes, that's right, the hospital food was amazing – if you can believe it), but I couldn't touch a thing.

'Can I eat it then?' he asked me. 'It looks gorgeous and I've had nothing all day.' Poor man, he was running himself ragged.

'Take it,' I urged. 'Don't forget to look after yourself – we are all going to need you!' I looked at the food and thought I was going to throw up.

While I was waiting to see the oncologist I wandered around the wards. There was a large children's section and I went in, attracted by the bright paintings and the sound of the *Jungle Book* soundtrack. It was full of children, but there was no shouting, no laughter. There was an eerie stillness in the ward. Some children were sitting watching a video; others were with their parents or looking at a book or a toy; some were just sitting by themselves staring into space. All were deathly pale and had knowing, old-man eyes. On later visits I would go in and chat to them, but that first day I backed out, horrified at the sight. Just looking at their small, sad faces brought tears to my eyes. What a cruel world, in which such suffering could happen to children so young and innocent.

Late that day the oncologist appeared. 'I'm sorry,' he said, 'we won't get the results until Monday. Why don't you go home for the weekend if you like, and come back in on Monday morning.'

'Is there anything we should do over the weekend?'

'Yes. Pray that it's Hodgkin's. That way you won't lose all your hair.'

I prayed that weekend as I had never prayed before.

Chapter Four

Loss and Relief

It was one of those rare glorious Irish weekends: the sky was cloudless and everyone was out enjoying the sunshine, leading normal family lives – as it seemed to us. For us it was the most unusual weekend we had ever lived through.

There is a photo of me taken that Sunday. I am sitting in the garden with Sarah on my knee. She looks gorgeous, full of life, her cheeky face framed by a brown bob. She is wearing one of the little outfits I had made for our holiday, which now seemed such an age ago. I look tired and strained – it's not the best picture of me I've ever seen – but we are both smiling at the camera. I remember so well looking at her that day, hugging her to myself and wondering if I would see her grow up.

We had decided that I would spend the Saturday and Sunday at home. After all, we reasoned, if I had a limited time ahead of me I should spend every possible moment with my children. The most important thing would be to act normally. 'Promise me this,' I said to Ger and his mother Anne, who had come to stay. 'Do not say anything that might make the children worry or suspect that something is amiss. No whispering, no quiet talking when they are around. We cannot discuss this at all.' I knew that Richard in particular was so close to me he would be bound to pick up on any snippets that we might let slip. They promised faithfully. I think for me, as well, it was important to try to carry on as usual. Ger was great, joking and laughing, full of humour and fun. There was an edge of desperation to his humour that weekend – he was trying to keep me going as if his life depended on it. And in a way, it did.

I felt then, more than ever, what a wise choice I had made in Ger. As I watched him chasing the children around the garden, wearing one of Richard's scary masks while Sarah screamed in mock terror, I cast my mind back to the night we met. We had been dancing that night, at the local rugby club do. It was the autumn of 1970, and I was sixteen.

One of my friends worked in a local record shop, and told me she had met two guys from Dublin earlier that day in the shop. They had told her they were staying the weekend in Drogheda and she had mentioned the rugby club dance. We both wondered if they would turn up, and sure enough, they did. Ger walked straight over to me and asked me to dance. He was nice-looking, with blond hair and blue eyes, and he had an open and friendly manner – not at all shy like many of the boys I had met. I was dark-haired, and very petite. I felt an instant attraction, and it was clear he did too. We danced together for the rest of the evening, but when it came to leaving I couldn't find him. I knew he lived in Dublin, the big city I longed to be part of, but as I lived in a small town some thirty miles away there was no way of contacting him. Well, I couldn't get him out of my head for months, and my chance came – or so I thought – when I went to see Thin Lizzy in Dublin at the National Stadium just before Christmas. Hardly paying attention to my favourite band, I scanned the audience again and again, checking every face, sure I would see him there. It wasn't the metropolis it is now of course, but even then I was crazy to think that I would find him at the gig. We left, my friend Catherine in high spirits singing 'Look What the Wind Blew In' at the top of her voice. I was dejected. More to the point, I thought, look what the wind *hadn't* blown in. 'Look Bernie,' she said, 'if it's to be, it will be.' We all set a lot of store by fate in those days.

I stayed with her that night, and the following day instead of going straight back to Drogheda we decided to go to the stock-car racing. It was good fun, and I knew Gerard was into it too. As we arrived, whom should we see leaving but Ger himself. My heart nearly stopped. Fate! I was beside myself – anxious to appear nonchalant, but desperate to talk to him. He came over to us (although we were pretending we hadn't seen him) and offered us a lift home. Naturally we accepted, although we had only just got there. He was driving his father's Rover and I admit I was impressed – the prospect of a boyfriend with a car would have turned any young girl's head at that time.

He dropped us off at home and my friend got out of the car and went in to talk to my mum. I stayed chatting with him – we got on well from the very first, and I was loath to leave him. When he mentioned he wanted some patches on his jeans – the height of fashion in the early seventies – I knew I had him. 'I could do that for you no problem,' I said easily. 'I'm good at sewing.' He asked me out that evening, and we're still together thirty-four years on.

He is my rock, as I needed no reminding that afternoon, watching him hold everything together for me and the family. His mother hadn't been so lucky, and nor had mine. The day wore on, dusk fell, and we all went in to put Richard and Sarah to bed.

'It's been a lovely day,' said Richard as I tucked him up. 'I'm glad you came back from hospital.' I sat on the edge of his bed and cupped his sweet, trusting face in my hands. I willed myself not to cry. 'It's been lovely for me too, Richard,' I whispered. 'But I may have to go back again soon.'

'Are you sick?' he asked.

'A little, yes, but I'll get better, don't you worry.'

'OK. Night, night.' He was so accepting, so sure that I was always going to be there. I prayed to God to protect my little boy from the pain and sorrow I feared was ahead.

As soon as the children were asleep that evening I burst into tears, unable to take the strain of trying to pretend everything was rosy any longer. The worry, the uncertainty, perhaps even the pregnancy hormones – all crowded in upon me, and I allowed all the emotions to flood out. I sobbed for a long time. Ger just held me in his arms, stroked my hair, and told me again and again that he loved me.

The next morning I woke up and found I was bleeding. I knew I was losing the baby now. I came out of the bathroom and called Gerard.

'I am sure I've lost the baby.' I said, trying to keep calm. He held my hand and comforted me. 'I'm sorry,' he said. 'Maybe it is for the best. It just isn't the right time.'

I wept, but with something like relief. This was God's way of helping me, I knew. I was overwhelmed with gratitude that I would not now be faced with making that cruellest of choices. I might recover from cancer but I would never recover from killing my own baby. I knew the memory would come back to haunt me for years. Even now I shudder to think about how close I was to the horror of that decision. This was just the way I felt, and no 'sensible' medical reasons could ever square that for me. Suddenly I thought of my mother, who had given birth to three stillborn babies – two between Jimmy and Aquinas, and one between Aquinas and Deirdre. Each time she came home from hospital and carried on as usual. It may have been more common in those days to lose a baby, and regarded as an unpleasant fact of life that one just had to deal with, but I cannot think that she did not grieve inwardly. I marvelled at her bravery and determination. If she could carry on after each successive loss, surely I could cope with the disappointment of this miscarriage.

'I'm fine, I really am,' I said briskly, getting dressed and readying myself to face the last day of not knowing.

Now I just had one thing to worry about – the cancer, which was looming large in front of us.

Chapter Five

The Diagnosis

~

'**O**h. Right,' was all the oncologist said the next day when I told him I had miscarried. He wasn't sympathetic, but nor was he unkind. To him it was simply a bald fact, and of course it removed a complication. He was doing his rounds at the time and told me he would have my results later in the day.

We waited in the ward all morning, sitting on two armchairs next to the same bed. There was not much to do other than watch the other patients, but what I saw shocked me to the core. The poor woman opposite me who had been so friendly on the Friday was unrecognizable. Out of her mind on morphine, she kept trying to get out of bed and was repeatedly helped back by the nurses. She was a little older than me, but in her I saw a vision of myself as I might become. It was a vision of hell. Frightened, I pulled the curtain around my bed and wept. *Please, God, can I not end up like her.*

'She has leukaemia, Bernie. You have got something else. You won't end up like that, trust me.' Ger busied himself with ordering prawn cocktail and steak and kidney pie, while I sat feeling nauseous at the very thought. The minutes seemed to stretch out endlessly, the hands on the large clock on the wall moving unbearably slowly.

'I keep thinking of Dad,' I told him. My recent dream was still with me, in the way that some dreams lurk at the sides of your consciousness, nagging at you, as if they are trying to tell you something. The smells of the hospital also reminded me of the last days I spent with him, and the grey, drawn faces of the patients on this ward brought back his dear, ravaged face clearly to me. Dad wasn't sick for long – he went downhill very quickly over two months, and I thought I'd heard somewhere that some cancers killed you quickly, while others lingered for years. Which kind would I be dealt, I wondered.

'I expect he's watching over you, you know. He may not have been at our wedding, but by God he loved his little girl.' I shut my eyes.

I had been twenty-five at the time, and due to be married to Ger that summer. We had been together for years but had been wary of rushing into marriage earlier: both sets of parents had been less than blissfully happy. But finally the wedding was all organized, the honeymoon booked. We were already living together: we couldn't afford to keep two flats going but this was something that was frowned upon in those days. I hadn't told my own mother – she hadn't asked, and I hadn't volunteered the information, but Ger's mother knew and was not at all happy about it. So we were quite keen to get on and marry. Then Dad got sick and everything changed.

I knew before I was told. One day I saw him walking up the hill to our house. He was only sixty-six but he was hunched over like a man twenty years older, coughing and coughing. He had been such an upright, smart man: he always wore a tie, his hair always neatly slicked back, even though he worked on construction sites. I knew there was something terribly wrong, and sure enough, a few days later he was in hospital for tests. Then he was sent home again, and when I asked my mother she seemed confused.

'I don't know, pet,' she said. 'I'll look after him here and let's hope he gets better.'

Ger collected me from work one day. 'I have some news for you about your Dad,' he said. 'He has cancer.' I needed to find out more, so I rushed in to the hospital to see the consultant. 'Can you tell me what's the story with my father?' I asked him. He explained that the tests were inconclusive, but he was fairly sure it was advanced cancer, and they would be doing more tests.

'Is he a smoker?' he asked.

'Yes,' I said. 'All his life. 80 Woodbines a day.' He made no reply, but shrugged his shoulders and held his palms up as if to say, 'Well, what can you expect?'

'I'm afraid there is very little that can be done for him at this stage. We will do our best to make him comfortable.'

Dad did not know he had cancer. It was a hushed word in those days, and still is, to a degree. It seems to be a taboo subject, second only to AIDS in the fear it inspires in people. I don't think we should be afraid of the word, and now I am very straight when I tell people what I have had. I regret now that I did not say, 'I know you're dying, tell me what you want to say.' I am sorry I did not tell him how much I loved him. But back then I was afraid too, and I was used to keeping secrets in my house.

'I want to walk you up the aisle, so I do,' my father said to me. 'Could you wait a little longer until I'm well?'

'Of course, Dad, we'll postpone it as long as we need to. You'll get better,' I promised.

But he was dead in two months. I could not save him.

The clatter of the dinner trolley brought me back to the present, and I looked up to see Ger rubbing his hands at the thought of the steak and kidney pie he had ordered. I could face nothing more than a cup of tea and slice of bread. We were both trying so hard not to fall to pieces, but the sinking feeling in the pit of my stomach refused to ease, even with a little food.

The afternoon ticked on. Shortly after the tea trolley had been round, the oncologist appeared. The moment of truth had arrived, and I splashed my tea on the bed cover in my hurry to stand up. I was surprised and immensely cheered – the man was beaming.

'Great news!' he announced. 'It's lymphoma. Cancer of the lymph glands.'

'Um – how is that great news?' I asked, glancing at Ger who was smiling broadly, if looking a bit confused.

'It is at a very early stage. You will not need chemotherapy, only steroids. You won't lose your hair. Nevertheless, you will be in and out of here over the next year or so.'

Suddenly I felt fantastic. I had spent the day believing that it was my fate to end up like the poor woman on the ward, or like my father. Now it appeared I was being given a stay of execution.

'You'll have a few more tests over the next few days, and then you'll need to take this prescription to the dispensary to collect your drugs. Follow the instructions on the packets. I'll get my secretary to make a follow-up appointment for a few weeks' time to see how you're getting on. Goodbye for now.' He shook our hands.

'Thank you, thank you,' I breathed, hugely grateful to this oncologist who, it seemed, had just told me I was not about to die after all. He was a hero, a saviour. A huge sense of relief washed over us both, and after he had gone we just stood there grinning stupidly at each other.

Later that day I had to have a piece of bone marrow taken out of my hip, I imagined so they could check to see whether the cancer had spread to the marrow. The doctor did not use an anaesthetic – I didn't think to ask why – but plunged the thick needle straight into my hip, twice, leaving it there each time for over a minute. I gasped in shock – I had never felt pain like this, and the only tools I had for dealing with agony like this were the breathing techniques I had learnt when I gave birth to Richard and Sarah. Holding on to a nurse I panted loudly, trying to rise above the pain and think of each breath. I squeezed her arm so tightly I must have hurt her quite badly. Then it was over.

The test results were clear, showing that – thankfully – the cancer had not spread. A few days later we walked through the ward on the way to the dispensary. The bed opposite mine was empty and I looked enquiringly at Ger. He put his arm around my shoulders. 'She's not in pain any longer.'

We left the hospital with mountains of drugs. The treatment had begun.

Chapter Six

Steroids: the Good ...

It was 2am and I was cleaning the house.

The kitchen was pristine, the bathrooms were shining. I crept into Sarah's room while she was sleeping, and reached up to the cupboards above her bed. They need to be sorted out, I decided, and I need to do it now. I put Richard's felt pens back in their boxes in neat colour-coordinated rows. I glanced at his toy soldiers, piled on a shelf in the playroom where he had chucked them that evening. That wouldn't do. Moments later they were all poised in position.

When Ger got up at 6am to go to work his breakfast was ready and I was dusting the living room. 'I feel so sorry for you,' he sympathized. 'You have been up all night.'

'Don't be sorry: I feel superb!' I countered. He laughed at me. 'You're my dream woman! I always wanted a wife who would keep the place spotless.'

'I don't know what's come over me,' I admitted. Normally I was a disaster in the house. I wasn't messy, but I wasn't particularly tidy either. I could exist with a certain amount of chaos around me – after all, that's what everyone's house is like if they have small children. I always felt it would drive me mad if I felt everything had to be perfect. But for some reason I had suddenly become filled with enormous energy and I had to channel it into something.

'Perhaps I'm going mad?' I suggested. I had never felt this compulsion to clean before. 'Look at those shoes.' I pointed to the shoe rack, where at least ten pairs of shoes were arranged in a smart rank, so shiny so you could almost see your face in them. Ger raised his eyebrows.

'Bernie – it's official. You're turning into your mother.'

My mother, Maria, was a tiny dynamo of a woman. She had grown up with her father and stepmother, who – as in the fairy tales – had two beloved children of her own. Mum was treated like a slave in her own home, and at the age of twelve she went into service like so many young girls in Ireland in the early 1920s. I remember hearing how she would have to get up at 4am to milk the cows, her fingers blue with cold, then she would go inside to lay the fires, break the ice on the wash stands, and work all day in the house without a break. When her tasks were finally over at around 11 at night, she would literally collapse into bed. She devoted her life to serving others, and when I and my four siblings were growing up in our small terraced house in Drogheda she would always be washing and scrubbing, cooking and cleaning –

never resting until the place was spotless. We were poor, but we were always well turned out. And our shoes, set out for us the night before school, were polished until they gleamed.

'Actually, I think it is the drugs.' I had been taking them for a few days and this huge burst of energy must be one of the side effects. The oncologist hadn't mentioned any side effects, so I dug out one of the packets and looked at the 'patient information leaflet'. Sure enough, there, in the midst of conditions I had never heard of like *promimal myopathy, Cushing's syndrome* and *negative nitrogen balance*, I found *euphoria, insomnia* and, more worryingly, *psychosis.*

'Well, perhaps I could take some to improve my golf swing,' Ger joked. 'I could do with some help.'

Not only was I behaving as if I wanted to win Housewife of the Year 1988, I was talking nineteen to the dozen. 'Slow down,' my garrulous friend Emma from down the road would say. 'Talk about gift of the gab. I can't keep up with you.' Yet I had to talk quickly to keep up with the speed at which my mind was going – I would be in the middle of a sentence and find myself already forming the next one. Life was going at 90 miles per hour. My brain raced with plans and schemes. I sat up late into the night, existing on very little sleep, making list after list. I still have these tucked away in a drawer, and I hardly recognize my writing – it is larger and more flamboyant than my usual restrained style. There are names of countries I wanted to visit for holidays; out-ings to take the children on; plans for redesigning the garden; things I thought we needed for the house; people I had lost touch with; books I wanted to read but could not sit still long enough to get through the first chapters. And all the while I was cleaning, cleaning, cleaning.

I had never taken mind-altering drugs, but I supposed this was what it was like for people who take coke, speed or ecstasy. 60mg of prednisone daily and I was on an absolute high. It felt fantastic. Everything was beautiful to me, colours were brighter, people were more attractive. And my children! I thought they were the most gorgeous creatures ever to have walked the earth. Everything I saw, everything I heard, everything I sensed was loaded with a meaning at once overwhelmingly powerful, and at the same time impossible to convey to anybody else. I was in my own private kingdom. And perhaps above all, I was able to make a difference, to make whatever I wanted happen.

One weekend we went to visit Ger's brother Paul and his wife Sharon. I was very excited and full of energy and conversation. I spent the whole time telling them how beautiful they were, how lovely the house was, and how much I loved them.

'Bernie, you're acting weird,' whispered Ger, taking me to one side. 'I know it seems normal to you, but remember these tablets you are on are making you behave a little differently.'

'OK, OK, I'll try not to say anything. But Ger,' I whispered back conspiratorially, 'don't you feel that things are getting better? I'm not going to die after all. I'm going to get better, and I have the loveliest family anyone could have. I'm so happy I could burst.'

He took me home early.

Friends and family flocked to our house. I invited them all, and they were keen to come. They had heard that I had been sick and could not believe how happy I was and how well I looked. I spent all day in the kitchen cooking for large numbers of people, serving up huge meals and wolfing mine down before anyone else. I would splash wine into people's glasses, not caring if it spilt. Even though I could not drink any myself while I was on medication I felt so high I might as well have been tipsy myself. It was the most wonderful feeling.

One day Emma brought a cake over. I gave it to the children after their tea and, as usual, most of it ended up on the floor. 'Never mind!' I said brightly. 'I'll clear it up.' Instead of fetching the dustpan and brush, though, I thought it was a perfectly good idea to crawl under the table on my hands and knees picking up each and every crumb. It took some time. 'You've gone stark raving mad,' said my friend, trying to stop me. 'Are you feeling OK? I thought you were meant to be ill.'

'What are you talking about?' I asked. 'I couldn't feel better.'

The next day I went to the garden centre with a very tall friend of mine, Helen. She bought two very heavy plants in large terracotta pots. I insisted on carrying them to the car. Again, she was horrified.

'Listen Bernadette, I'll do that. Don't go making yourself sick again by lugging things like this around. At least let me take one.'

'Don't be silly, I'm fine. I need to carry on as normal, Helen. Don't fuss.' I grabbed the plants and staggered off. It must have looked comic, though, to anyone watching. Me, a diminutive five feet tall, dwarfed by these two huge plants, accompanied by Helen who towers above me by almost a foot.

Then one day I woke up and couldn't move my arms.

Chapter Seven

... the Bad ...

I couldn't understand it – the previous day I had been fine. Now I simply couldn't raise my arms. My elbows were stiff and unbending, agony when I tried to move them. Was I paralysed? No, I could move the rest of my body, although my legs hurt. Why had I suddenly seized up? Was this the lymphoma or was this another side effect of the steroids? No one had warned me of this. Ger had already left the house for work, and I could hear the children stirring in their rooms. They would be getting themselves dressed and needing breakfast in a few minutes. What was I to do? Come on Bernie, I said to myself, you can work out a way to get out of bed without your arms. I couldn't sit up, and I found my knees were painful to bend too so I couldn't use them to propel myself. Eventually I managed to roll onto my side and slide out of bed, but when I put pressure on my knees I collapsed. They were like jelly.

I sat on the floor by the bed. This was bad. The children were arguing about something and I heard a door being slammed. I had three things to do: 1: Stand up; 2: make breakfast; 3: take them to school. At that moment these three things seemed like the hardest tasks anyone could ask of me. I couldn't imagine how

I was going to get through the first half hour of today, let alone the rest of it.

I half stood up, gritting my teeth against the pain. The phone was on the bedside table, and I managed to lean my body over to pick it up. I called Gerard.

'I can't move,' I whispered, 'All my joints have seized up. I don't know what to do.' I explained how long it had taken me to get up and how worried I was.

'Will I come home?' he offered. 'Or will I call Pauline for you?'

Pauline was a neighbour, and had a lad at the same junior school as Richard and Sarah. Over the course of the next few months I would have cause to thank God for Pauline many times.

'I'll try her. Don't you worry for now. I might be feeling better later; I'll see how it goes.' I needed to hear Ger's voice, but I didn't want to worry him too much. I already felt better for talking to him.

'OK, but will you call me to let me know? Oh, and try the hospital too – they might be able to help.'

'Yes I will. See if you can come home a little early though. Bye.'

Then I remembered the information leaflet in the prednisone box by my bed. I shook it out of the box and read it. Sure enough, there was an extensive list of side effects, including something they described as *muscle weakness* or *joint pain*. Was that it? It made no mention of excruciating agony – how odd. How typical.

With great effort I got myself downstairs, calling the children on my way. I persuaded them that it would be fun for them to get out the breakfast things and pour out their own milk and orange juice this morning. While it saved me from reaching into cupboards it did not make for an entirely mess-free kitchen, and when I looked in on them after calling Pauline to ask her to take them to school my heart sank to see the spilt cereal and puddles of milk dripping onto the floor. They were both giggling. I knew then that I would have to stay cheerful for their sakes.

'Never mind,' I said to them. Some of my standards were just going to have to slip.

After I had gratefully sent them both off with Pauline I collapsed onto the sofa. The pressure on my knees from having been up for three quarters of an hour had left them aching more than before and I needed to raise them up. I called the hospital as soon as I thought there would be someone there to answer.

'Oh, don't worry, Mrs Bohan,' said the nurse in a reassuring voice. 'That is just one of the side effects of this drug – there are various different ones and everyone reacts differently. The cortisone does reach the joints and can cause some discomfort.'

Discomfort? I managed a rueful smile. I still had the leaflet tucked in my pocket and my hand shook as I scanned the list for other symptoms. *Abdominal pain, acne, allergic reactions...*

increased appetite, hair growth, nausea, fluid retention, osteoporosis, indigestion, depression, headaches, hallucinations, insomnia... I stopped reading. I knew if I continued I would start imagining I had all these side effects. Tackle one thing at a time, I decided.

Over the next few days the cortisone seeped through to every joint in my body, right through to my fingers and toes. I learnt that the only way to lead anything approaching a normal life would be to pace myself carefully. I was in unbelievable pain when I woke up each morning, my joints stiff and immovable. Richard and Sarah were always taken to school by my neighbour – I would be literally hunched over like an old crone, and in no state to go anywhere at that time of day. I would gradually loosen up until I could almost stand upright, which would be around midday. I was never able to stand completely straight, and this in itself put a huge strain on my back. At half past one I had pulled myself together sufficiently to be ready to leave the house to collect the children, but I would shuffle up the road at no more than a snail's pace. For everyone else it took just six minutes; for me it took over half an hour. Then we would potter back home, the children skipping back and forth along the pavement like puppies, covering three times the distance I travelled in half the time.

Household tasks – as few as I could reduce them to – I would spread throughout the day, and I did as many as I could sitting down, so as not to strain my knees too much. Anything extra, anything enjoyable – like gardening, or sewing – was out of the question. This was so strange for me: even before my recent period of hypomanic behaviour, I was not a person for sitting around. I like to be up and about, busy and active. I have no patience for lounging about and I hardly ever watch television. What a punishment this was for me! It drove me mad not to be able to do things, particularly when I knew how much there was to get done. Perhaps this was God's way of telling me to slow down – I often think that He finds ways of teaching us the lessons we most need to learn.

I was taking sixteen prednisone tablets each day, plus one Tagamet to prevent stomach ulcers. I took the first dose early in the morning, and then at four hour intervals throughout the day. About half an hour after I'd taken the tablets I would feel an easing of the pain, and I would be relatively fine for the next two hours, after which the pain would return and I would find myself counting the minutes until the allotted time for the next dose. The periods of lesser pain were when I would schedule any tasks I had to do – I paced my own activities to match the rhythms of the drugs. I also knew I couldn't be on my feet too much or for too long, or I'd pay for it with excruciating pain later.

One afternoon I was up at the school waiting for the children. I put on a bright smile to greet the other mothers who clustered around the school gates. I noticed the mother of one of Richard's friends looking at me curiously. Marian knew I had been ill, and asked me how I was doing.

'Not so good, if I'm honest,' I replied. This wasn't like me. I hardly ever talked to anyone about how I was feeling, apart from Ger, but I knew she would understand the situation because she was a nurse. She might even have some ideas on how I could help myself. 'These steroids are giving me pain in my joints like I've never known, and I'm wondering what I can do to ease the pain. Do you think maybe I should bring forward the times at which I take them, like take them every three hours instead of every four?'

'No, definitely not, don't be tempted to do that,' she warned. 'If you did that you would effectively be increasing your dose. Take paracetamol in between doses to keep the pain down – and take the maximum dose it allows on the packet. You might also try bandaging your joints tightly – that should help.'

I followed her advice gratefully. I learnt to take the paracetamol around half an hour before the time I estimated the pain would be at its peak, so I was able to cope until the next dose of prednisone. The nights were the worst. My mind was still racing as it had during the first three crazy weeks, but my body was shutting down. I craved sleep because it was the only time I was pain-free, yet I would rarely drift off for longer than an hour or so at a time, so I was dropping with weariness during the day. Ger used to bandage my knees tightly before we went to bed, and I found the pressure did relieve the pain a little.

'Why don't you think about taking something to help you to sleep?' Ger urged me.

'No, I'm taking so many tablets already. I hate all these drugs – if there is something I can do without I think I should try, don't you?' Of course he agreed. Ger was incredibly supportive and would have done anything to try to help ease my suffering, yet he knew how strongly I always had felt about taking medication.

He felt guilty for waking me in the night, for even if I did manage to drop off I would wake instantly if he turned over, coughed or snored. Eventually we had to sleep in separate rooms. This was sad for both of us – it was the only time in our lives when we have slept apart. Yet it meant that I was able to snatch perhaps one hour's extra sleep.

'Goodnight, sleep well,' we would whisper to each other on the landing outside the children's bedrooms. We would stand for a while with our arms round each other, Ger holding me so gently in order not to bruise me. I had never needed comfort and closeness more, yet I had never felt so cut off from normal human contact. I was full of bitterness. Only a few months ago I had been so happy and carefree. Now I could not imagine feeling worse.

'God, how I hate this. I hate the drugs, I hate the pain, I hate not being able to lead a normal life. I hate moping around the house feeling useless.'

'Just remember that these drugs are helping you,' he would keep saying. 'This won't last for ever.'

'That's what the oncologist says,' I responded grumpily. I was seeing him every month, and each time he would check the size of the lump, as well as checking my neck, my stomach and under my arms, for there was the constant fear that the cancer would surface elsewhere. While he did this I would fire question after question at him, desperate to understand the disease and find ways of helping myself. On one visit when I was chatting to (Gerard would say interrogating) one of the nurses she shook her head at me. 'Books? You don't want to go there – you will only end up frightening yourself.' I realized years later that that was the worst piece of advice anyone ever gave me. Now, when I teach people about health I always tell them that knowledge is power – get informed, educate yourself, get some control.

The oncologist could not recommend any books either. He always said I was responding well to the treatment – the lump was shrinking – but sometimes I suspected he was just trying to make me feel better. I was to be on the drugs for several months. If I thought things couldn't get worse, I was wrong.

Chapter Eight

... and the Ugly

'There she is,' Richard pointed at me. 'I told you she was fat. Look at her.'

It was true. I was parked on the sofa one afternoon watching television, trying not to put pressure on my knees. Richard, just home from school, had brought three of his friends over to see me. They all stared open-mouthed at me for a moment, then rushed out to play in the garden. I smiled ruefully to myself – I had become a freak show for my kids. I knew all these lads, and they knew me. I didn't blame Richard for showing me to them like this – after all I *was* fat. It was horrific to me, but just a fact of life to him. I had changed, and there it was. Even Sarah had taken to calling me her 'fat Mammy'.

I am short, with a small frame, and I normally weigh around 45 kilos, or seven and a half stone. I had heard that people could put on weight with steroids, and the last thing I wanted to do was to acquire the physique of an Eastern Bloc shot-putter. But since that July, when I started taking prednisone, I had been ravenous. Even after a huge meal I would still be hungry and I was constantly fighting the urge to binge. Although I was aware of eating healthily and always tried to be careful, I quickly did put on weight – muscle weight, as well as fat weight. It was hard, rock hard, like a layer of cement under my skin. My stomach looked engorged, almost pregnant. My neck was thick, solid with a mass of hard tissue. My face was so swollen I could hardly see the television. My ankles were huge and my shoes no longer fitted me. Within two months of starting the treatment my whole body had swollen up like a balloon. I could not look in the mirror without crying.

'I've never made love to a fatty before,' said Ger, trying to make me laugh. 'Your boobs are gorgeous.' He did make me feel better, and I was determined not to let my hideous shape affect the way I behaved. I believed that these drugs were making me well again and I wanted to live much, much more than I wanted to be thin again. So I still shuffled up the hill to collect the children and tried to ignore the looks from people who didn't know me. It did hurt when people I knew fairly well would cross the road rather than speak to me, and I kept telling myself that it was because they were embarrassed and did not know what to say to me.

I did get out when I could, and not just to the school gates. I went shopping in my 'good' periods, just down to the local supermarket. As I handed the groceries to the cashier one day, who was a girl I knew quite well, she looked up at me in surprise.

'Jesus, what happened to your face?' The words were out before she realized how appalling they sounded. She clapped her hands over her mouth and looked stricken.

'I'm on medication right now,' was all I could manage.

'I'm so sorry,' she called after me. 'I didn't mean ...'

I got home somehow, and shut the door behind me. Safe once more, I leaned against it and decided never, ever to go into that shop again. I don't think of myself as a vain person. I look OK, that's all, and I don't bother with make-up every time I go out – a slick of lippy normally does the trick for me. But to feel truly ugly, that is a different matter. My face was round, moon-shaped. I thought I looked like a giant chipmunk.

One morning we had a parents' meeting at the school to discuss our children's work. I dressed carefully, taking care with my appearance as much as I could, for I always liked the children to be proud of me. The meeting took place in Sarah's classroom, and while I was waiting I occupied myself with looking at the brightly coloured artwork on the walls. I was the next one to be seen, and Sarah's teacher looked up at me and then down at her list. 'I'm sorry,' she said, extending her hand and introducing herself. 'You must be, ah, Sarah's aunt?' My heart stopped.

'No, actually I'm her mother, but I'm on medication at the minute,' I managed to blurt out.

'I'm terribly sorry,' she stammered, clearly embarrassed by her mistake. Somehow we both got through the meeting, which was not easy since at that time Sarah was not doing too well at school,

71

and I blamed myself for not being able to give her enough attention at home. As I left the school, tears were rolling down my cheeks. My own child's teacher doesn't recognize me, I thought. Will I ever look normal again? I didn't see one of the other mothers coming towards me and, disorientated, I almost walked into her. 'Are you OK?' she asked, seeing my distress. I didn't know her well, but I knew her name was Patricia. It was one of those moments when virtual strangers can be of more help than close friends, and I told her everything.

I went out less and less, and persuaded some of the other mothers to drop off the kids for me so I did not have to face the world. I felt more and more isolated. Of course I had Gerard, and I had the children, but I still felt terribly alone. The days were awfully long, at home by myself. I didn't have many friends nearby at that stage, as we hadn't been in the house very long and I was only just starting to meet people through school. I had no close girlfriend to confide in apart from Marian.

'This won't go on for ever,' she kept saying. 'Just hang on in there.'

'Oh, look at this will you now,' I cried one day, after discovering to my horror a thick covering of downy hair on my top lip. I was growing a moustache, and my natural hair colour was dark brown. Any day now Gerard was going to start calling me Hitler.

'Now don't you go fretting over that, Bernadette. Just bleach it and no one will notice. Whatever you do, don't shave it. Leave it be and when all this is over you'll be back to normal with no harm done.'

I had not told my mother that I had cancer. She was in her seventies and becoming frailer by the day, so I felt that news such as this would crush her. I did not want her to worry – what good would that have done anyone? And it might just finish her off: I could not face losing her on top of everything else. My sister Aquinas had just had a new baby after losing one, so the last thing I wanted was to upset her. I was the baby of the family and had always been a bit spoilt and treated special. I knew that it would shock them all to the core to think that I was in mortal danger – it would have been against the normal order of things for me to have a fatal illness before the others. So I battened down the hatches, kept quiet, and tried my best to get through each day.

'Bernie,' said Gerard one evening. 'Have you remembered what's coming up at the end of the month?'

'Oh!' I gasped. 'August 21st!' I had completely forgotten. The end of August was always celebrated in our family. It marked both the anniversary of my father's death and Richard's birthday, and we always got together for a family day and a bit of a party. There was no way I could get out of it. Mum in particular always looked forward to the day and would spend days preparing food for all of us. Since my father's death she had really come out of herself – she had her own freedom at last and was enjoying life to the full. A few days before the party I called my mother to have a chat about the day – of course, my main reason for this was to prepare her a little. I mentioned to her that I was on tablets and looked a bit swollen. But nothing could prepare her for the shock of seeing me in the flesh.

She gave a little scream when she saw me. 'Bernadette, will you look at your face? What has happened to you? I hardly recognize my own daughter.'

'I told you, Mum, I'm on some tablets at the minute.'

'Well, we'll just have to get you off them, that's all. You tell your doctor they're not doing you any good – they're destroying you.' And that, as far as she was concerned, was that. She was always very protective of me, being her youngest.

When Aquinas saw me she burst into tears. 'Sweet Jesus, Bernie, what's wrong?' I couldn't not tell her.

'It's cancer,' I whispered, not wanting Mum or the kids to hear, 'but the treatment is working. I know I look bad, but it's for the best. Don't you worry, I'll be fine.' She nodded, aghast, as I explained about the lymphoma and the steroids. I tried to make light of it – I couldn't see her upset, because even though she is my older sister I wanted to protect her. Thankfully my other sister Deirdre could not make it that day – she is a big softie and I knew she would find it hard to deal with. It was a strange day, most unlike all the other end-of-August parties we had held. Gerard and I were putting a brave face on things, Aquinas kept shooting me pitying glances, and my mother kept telling us all that I looked a fright. Even the kids were jumpy – they picked up the air of unreality and uncertainty. Cancer was back in all our lives once more, and it was to change everything.

When we left, some time later, we drove through the town and passed Aquinas standing talking to a friend. She was crying her eyes out. I felt sorry she was upset, but relieved that at last I had been able to tell her.

And so the days wore on, the weeks turned into months, and I got better at dealing with the pain and facing my reflection in the mirror. On good days I would feel cheered that I had managed to cook a meal, or do some painting after school with the children. On bad days I would wonder if I would ever come out of this intact. I felt like a monster, like a mistake of nature, and I would seethe with anger. One evening some old friends came over. I love them both dearly, but they had no idea how they upset me that night. I watched them sit together on the sofa, him stroking her thigh as if she needed polishing. I was furious. How dare they do that in front on me? I raged inwardly. They looked so perfect, beautiful, whole; and I was hideous, swollen and sore. Get out of here and do it in your own house, I thought. I needed this like a hole in the head. In my raw anger I could not see that they had come to see me in a spirit of kindness and only meant well. It seemed to me that they were there to gloat, and to have a good look at me in my wretchedness. That's how twisted my view of everything had become.

The final few weeks were intolerable. In late October I went back to the oncologist for my monthly appointment. My face was so puffy and swollen I could barely see out of the slits of my eyes. He looked up as I entered the room and a look of sharp surprise crossed his face. He held up his hands as if I was about to shoot him.

'I'm taking you off them! I'm taking you off them!' he said.

I was full of gratitude and relief. This man had saved my life. He had treated me, I was better, and now he was saving me from the treatment itself. He told me I could come off them straightaway, and I left his surgery feeling elated. It was over. I was cured of the cancer and I could now go back to a normal life. I stopped taking the steroids that very day.

What a mistake that was.

The next morning I woke up shivering, feverish, by turns boiling hot or freezing cold, rigid with shock. My body was suffused with pain, and I had vomiting bouts. I felt panicked.

'Do something Ger, I'm frightened,' I begged.

'I'll call the doctor straightaway,' he said.

'No. Don't do that. Ring Marian.'

It was only later that I understood I'd been going through withdrawal symptoms more suited to a heroin addict than an ordinary mother-of-two. Marian's father had had leukaemia and had been on the same drug as me for some time. She would know what was going on.

'What do you mean she has just stopped taking it? That's crazy, you can't stop a drug like prednisone abruptly. She needs to wean herself off it gradually. Very gradually. Let me talk to her.'

Marian explained that I should go back to the full dose. I felt as if I had been promised a ticket to Heaven and now told that I should go straight back to Hell.

'No, Marian, please, I can't stay on those drugs a day longer.' She must have heard the disappointment in my voice.

'You have to, Bernadette. Your body will go into shock otherwise – it messes with your adrenal system something horrible. You must give your body a chance to adjust and it can't do it overnight. You've been taking sixteen tablets a day. Go back to sixteen, then in three days take it down to fifteen. Stay on fifteen for three days, then reduce to fourteen, and so on.' We worked out a schedule, and it took me many weeks to come off them completely. I thanked her so many times, but I suspect Marian will never know how much of a life-saver she was to me.

The joint pain finally receded. The hard muscle weight faded away. I looked like my old self again, and I was thrilled.

'Let's have a treat today,' said Gerard one Saturday shortly after I had finished coming off the drugs. 'What would you really like to do?'

'What I really fancy is some new clothes,' I said, feeling as excited as a little girl.

'Right then, come on you lot, let's go,' said Gerard. We all piled into the car and went into Dublin. What a wonderful day we had, the four of us, wandering around the city, choosing new clothes for me. I revelled in my new body, loving the chance to feel like a real woman again after months of being a freak. Sarah was great, making me try on everything, running around the shops pulling clothes off racks she thought I'd like. It reminded me of the feeling you get when you have just had a baby, or just stopped breastfeeding, and you are starting afresh with a new wardrobe. I still have a khaki suit and blouse from Principles I bought that day – it was so smart, and I felt so good in it.

But the best part was giving away all the clothes I had worn during that terrible time. I felt like I was throwing the year away. I was better, and nothing would stop me now.

Chapter Nine

New Life

Gradually I tried to put the cancer behind me, to banish it to the dark places of my mind. It was a blip, a freak event, I told myself. The treatment had been shattering, but it had worked. I had come through it, I was cured. Wasn't I here to prove it? I was feeling terrific, going to the gym, eating well (or so I thought), and – most importantly – throwing myself back into the job of being a mother, relishing its humdrum tedium as much as the sudden flashes of pure joy. Sarah was six and Richard was eight, and Ger was working hard. My life settled down and took on a certain familiar routine: housework, preparing meals, walking the children to school and collecting them, tidying up around them, helping them with their work, drying their tears, kissing their bumps and bruises better, sharing their small triumphs and disasters, ferrying them to parties and after-school activities. Richard went to tennis lessons and played football seemingly non-stop; Sarah was passionate about art, drama and tap dancing.

All this and more made up the delightful monotony of domestic life. In any spare moments I'd be at my sewing machine, running up clothes for them and for friends. It was something I enjoyed, and I felt it was so important for me to be in the home, always there for the kids if they needed me. At the weekends we would visit one of my sisters, or my mother, or one of Ger's family. We were a family who talked and laughed all the time, very sociable, very close. With so many of us there was always a reason to celebrate something – a birthday, a driving test passed, an anniversary. These were very special times: I loved every moment, knowing it was all the more precious to me because I had been so close to losing it all. Not a day went by without my sinking to my knees and thanking God for saving me for my children. They were so young, so vulnerable, so innocent in their trust that I would always be there. I used to slip into their bedrooms while they slept and stand for long moments watching over them, marvelling at their smooth unblemished skin and their sweet childish faces.

Don't imagine by this that I became some kind of perfect, self-less paragon of motherhood. No, we had our share of arguments and shouting matches, and they would test my patience to the limits. I would yell at them to brush their teeth, tidy their rooms, get in the car. At times they fought like cat and dog – I always seemed to be splitting up rows, and 'Stop it, the two o'you!' became a constant refrain. We were a normal family doing normal things. But at the same time I had such a sharp sense of the closeness of loss, the knowledge that we stand on a knife edge between happiness and sorrow. I was determined to surround them with as much love and care as I myself had been surrounded with by my own mother all those years before – a love that had given me such a strong sense of myself and had set such an example of selfless giving.

Meanwhile my oncologist was checking me and checking me. I thought I was cured; he was waiting for the cancer to come back.

What I did not know then was that once you have suffered from cancer you stand a much higher chance of getting it back, no matter how well you have responded to treatment. For the first three years after the lymphoma had disappeared, I checked myself constantly, obsessively, ever-vigilant for a sign that the cancer was returning. My appointments were scheduled for every three months for the first few years, then – the relief – every six months – a clear sign that I was doing well. We couldn't relax completely, of course, for according to him my lymphoma had been very rare and we had no statistics to go by. However, in between the appointments I would throw myself back into the business of living with the sort of determination and vigour I had seen in my mother all those years ago. There was so much going on in my children's lives I hardly had a chance to think about myself – indeed, I was reluctant to dwell on my own problems, knowing that the past has a habit of springing up to grab you when you least expect it. While the knowledge of what I had been through was always there, I was stubbornly keeping it at bay.

But I will never forget those regular hospital appointments. As I entered the hospital and walked down the sterile corridor to the familiar waiting room I felt as if I had never left, and all the old feelings would come flooding back. In this waiting room I might meet a woman wearing a wig, or a man whose stick-thin figure and gaunt cheeks spoke volumes. There but for the grace of God, I would think, feeling so sorry for them, but glad it was not me.

'Hello there,' I would chirrup to my oncologist, once in the consulting room, my false cheeriness covering my nerves. 'How are things?' We would chit-chat about holidays, the kids, or Ger. Then I would take off my clothes and lie down on the bed while he examined me all over, checking and re-checking my groin, back, breasts and underarms for anything sinister. Sometimes I asked him to check my glands if I thought they were swollen; or another part of me where I might have felt something a few days earlier. I would stare at his face, trying to read his mind, imagining that I could decipher my fate from the twist of his mouth or the slight frown on his forehead. I often found myself holding my breath until he said, 'Get dressed again Bernadette, you're fine.'

'Are you sure now, are you quite sure?' Relief, each time, blessed relief, flooded through me as he smiled his confirmation. And it was then that I would ask my question.

'Can I have another baby?'

He fixed me with his gaze – kind but unbending. 'No, Bernadette. No you can't. As you know, I think your lymphoma may have been activated by the pregnancy hormones. There is quite a bit of evidence suggesting this may be the case. We don't know for sure, but you simply cannot risk it. You'd be mad to give up everything you have now, everything you have survived for. Put it out of your mind – you already have two lovely children – a boy and a girl – and that is more than most people have. Go home and live your life.'

This was his standard answer. Pregnancy might kick-start the cancer again. Cancer could kill me. Having another baby could tear my family apart. I knew he would shake his head and intone the same deadpan response each time I saw him, but each time I knew I would have to ask him the same question. I was obeying an inner compulsion sharper than hunger; stronger than desire. My head told me I was foolish to imagine I could have another child, yet my heart longed for a baby.

For seven years I never gave up hoping that one day he'd 'give me permission'. I prayed that there would be some new scientific discovery – some new drug perhaps – that would enable me to carry a child to term without making myself sick or losing the baby. I was desperate for someone with a PhD to claim that pregnancy never triggered the growth of cancer cells. Or I needed a test to prove that my kind of cancer was caused by something entirely different.

I think it is something that anyone who has lost a baby will understand, that yearning to fill the empty place the unknown baby should have filled. How I wondered about that lost child: who it would have looked like, how it would have been with three children running around. I came from a large family – it was a natural thing for me to expect a big family for myself. I liked to think of him or her as my special guardian angel who had been with me for such a short time, giving me hope and comfort in the dark days of fear as I waited for the diagnosis, then quietly taking its leave of me to allow me, eventually, to be healed. Some people believe that children choose their parents – that they are souls that come to us to fulfil a need in us as much as in them. I don't know about this, but I did believe that it was all part of God's purpose, and who was I to question it?

Not that I was obsessed, you understand. I wasn't depressed, I wasn't crazy, I wasn't about to rob another woman of her child if I saw it in a pram in the supermarket. I felt nothing approaching the way friends of mine who have been trying unsuccessfully for a baby for many years feel. In the same way that I had learned to live with cancer, accept it, and take what good I could from the experience, I learned to live with this loss. The void would always be there, and the space I had set aside in my heart for another child was simply a fact of life. I took out all of Sarah's pretty little baby and toddler clothes which I had carefully packed away for a younger sibling. I held them to my cheek and inhaled what was left of her babyhood, mourning my lost third child who would never wear them. Then I washed and ironed them and gave them away. Toys and books that were gathering dust, never to be held by the chubby little fingers of a child of mine again – they all went too. After all, how could I jeopardize the life that I had fought so hard to keep? No, I knew I had to move forward, embrace life with outstretched arms and enjoy what I was so fortunate to have been given. Ger was happy as we were, and was anxious for me not to worry about having another baby. 'Look, love, put it out of your mind – it's not going to happen. Don't rock the boat.' I knew this was right, and sometimes I would give myself little pep talks: 'Come on Bernie now, get a grip. You're doing fine. Your kids are doing fine. You don't need another child.' I reluctantly accepted that it was not to be. But the want never disappeared.

So I got on with living my life, as women do. With so much going on in the house with my young children I couldn't mope around, and besides I'm a real doer – I hate sitting around doing nothing.

In May 1994 we had four weddings to go to: one was a family wedding and the others were colleagues of Ger's. Each weekend there would be another long drive, another traditional Irish knees-up where we had great craic, as they say. A good laugh, a great time. I always enjoy weddings – they are so full of life – and I suppose I must have been extra-relaxed after one of these occasions. I remember seeing all the small kids running around and I held the baby of a friend while she got up and danced. The little thing looked into my eyes and gave a big toothless grin, and my heart melted. The need for another child wasn't vague and formless any more, it was an ache I couldn't assuage. I had a strong feeling that somewhere out there was a child waiting in the wings for me to be its mother. That night I chose to embrace my destiny.

I wasn't on the Pill as I had had cancer, so we followed what I call the 'temperature' method of natural family planning. This system enables you to become attuned to your own time of ovulation – the few days around which you are most likely to become pregnant and should avoid intercourse. When Ger took me in his arms that night I murmured to him that I hadn't taken my temperature that day, and I knew it was around the middle of the month. 'I really want a baby,' I remember saying softly, and he simply replied, 'Let's not get into that now, love.'

A few weeks later we were in Cork for a couple of days' holiday with the children. We did a little sightseeing and swimming – it was a lovely break. When the kids were busy one afternoon on the beach I decided it was time to tell Ger my period was late. 'You've been late before, haven't you?' he asked, without missing a beat. That was true; a few days here and there never bothered me. This was different though – this was more than a few days. We sat holding hands looking out at the choppy sea, contemplating the enormity of the prospect. Neither of us really believed it could be happening.

A few days later I sat in the bathroom at home with a pregnancy test. It was one of those Plus and Minus kits, where a plus sign equals baby and a minus sign equals no baby. My heart was in my mouth. I was excited and fearful at the same time. As I stared at it, slowly but surely a small cross appeared. I was pregnant. The little cross seemed like a tiny sign of hope. 'What God takes away he gives back in His own good time' – my mother's words came back to me. I sat there for a long time.

I didn't know whether to laugh or cry. Part of me was elated – I had done it! We had been given the chance to have another child! But part of me was imploding with dread. The cancer. It might bring the cancer back. My oncologist would be furious. I imagined the progesterone coursing through my body, doing its job of thickening the lining of my womb and providing a nourishing place for my baby to grow, but at the same time being the evil poison that might somehow trigger the unnatural cell division that causes cancerous tumours to grow. This sweet promise of life that simultaneously held the threat of death.

When Ger came home that evening he had hardly put his things down before asking the question: 'So – plus or minus, Bernie? Was it plus or minus?' We were talking in code and the children looked up in surprise. Were we discussing a maths test or something? 'Plus!' I grinned, unable to conceal my delight. 'It's a plus!'

'Oh my God,' said Ger, wide-eyed and managing a smile, 'this is going to change our lives.' That had to be the understatement of the decade, I thought.

We didn't tell Sarah for a while, but Richard found out by accident a few days later. He was off school the day I went to see the GP in order to have the pregnancy officially confirmed with a urine test, so that was that secret well and truly out in the open. I took him off to a coffee shop for lunch and the little lad could not contain his excitement – he could hardly sit still. Leaping ahead as children do, he kept exclaiming, 'A brother! Mum, I'll be able to show him how to play football!' I couldn't dampen his childish enthusiasm, but I did try to explain that because mummy had been sick things might not always go to plan. 'Steady, son, I lost a baby once before, you know. Don't get carried away now.'

Dear God, please don't let me lose this baby, I prayed, please don't take it away from us. I had to hang on to it, I had to stay well.

While my family wanted to celebrate, my doctor made an appointment for me to see the oncologist as soon as possible.

He looked up at me when I entered his surgery. Because it was an unscheduled appointment he knew that there could only be two reasons for my appearance. Either the cancer was back, or I was pregnant. Or both. He looked at the file on his desk containing the referral letter from my GP. Wordlessly he motioned me to lie on the couch. This felt totally different from my normal appointments. No friendly banter, no routine questions and answers. It was only a couple of months since he had given me, for the enth time, his 'don't even think of getting pregnant' spiel. Yet I was desperate for a word of reassurance, something to make me believe it was all going to be OK. He checked me for any signs that the cancer was 'presenting'. Nothing. 'You're fine.'

At the moment.

I waited for him to rail at me for my temerity in getting pregnant, but he just looked unbearably weary. He wasn't going to tell me to get rid of the baby; he knew well enough how much I wanted it. Instead, he said brusquely but not unkindly, 'You're back in the system now. You'll be in and out of here throughout your pregnancy.'

So I was a 'cancer patient' again. I had been doing all right – well, even – and now I wasn't.

He put his hand on my shoulder as I rose to leave. 'Poor Bernadette,' he murmured.

Chapter Ten

'A Little Miracle'

My heart sank as I left the hospital. Like any woman who wants a child, I had been rejoicing in my pregnancy, despite the nagging worry. Now the oncologist had struck fear into my heart. Here I was, defiantly, stupidly pregnant, after so many warnings to put all thoughts of a baby out of my mind. I knew from his comments seven years before that his main priority would be to keep me well, and I remembered as if it was yesterday his workaday reaction to my last miscarriage. I wondered if he was hoping I would miscarry again. It would certainly make his life easier: one fewer potential cancer patient to treat.

Bernie, I said to myself, you've done it now. There's no going back. This is a baby you have wanted for so long – you are risking everything for it. It dawned on me that in the eyes of the medical establishment I was being irresponsible; but for me I was obeying a compulsion stronger than sense. It may not have been a rational, sensible, thought-through choice, but it was a deep and instinctive biological and emotional need. It was a decision I had made with my heart and soul. He thought I was mad, yet I had never felt saner.

Despite this inner conviction that I was somehow doing the right thing for me, for my family and for my unborn child, I was sick with worry. My body was changing by the day, and these changes – fascinating as they had been during my previous pregnancies – now brought with them new fears. Were my breasts sore and lumpy because of the pregnancy hormones, or could I feel a new tumour in its early stages? Was the pain in my lower back normal or sinister? Was I tired because my body was working overtime to establish the pregnancy, was I exhausted from trying to look after two young children, or could this be the first sign of lymphoma returning? I fretted constantly about losing the baby, and every time I went to the bathroom I told myself not to be surprised if I was bleeding. However, when the morning sickness started around the fifth week, I began to believe that this little embryo was really there, making its presence felt, and I felt a small shiver of pleasure through my anxiety and nausea.

I didn't talk about it to the children. Richard seemed to have forgotten for now, and since I showed no outward signs of being pregnant, Sarah was not aware of anything.

They were at each other in those first few weeks though more than ever, and it seemed as if I was constantly breaking up fights. Maybe I was less involved with them, perhaps I left them to their own devices more than usual. Certainly I was wrapped up in myself and my fears, and I know how my moods can affect them. I would wake up each morning, throw up, then have a shower, running my hands over my body – checking for any signs that the cancer was back. Once dressed, I would put on my Happy

Mummy face, have some dry toast for breakfast and get the kids ready for school. It was only when I returned home that I would sink into a chair and weep. I was so full of dread, so afraid that my pregnancy would bring back the cancer. It was as if a dark shadow was waiting in the wings to envelop me. It felt so close I could almost reach out and touch it.

Gerard kept me going through those first few weeks like never before. I cannot put a number on the times I would call him at work and offload my worries of the day. He always had time to listen, and always offered some reassuring words.

'Bernie, don't forget that the first few weeks of any pregnancy are like a rollercoaster. You've got all those hormones whizzing around your body. They are bound to make you feel more emotional than usual.'

'I know that's true, but these are the very hormones that might trigger the lymphoma again.'

'Listen, we don't know that for definite. It has always been something the doctors thought was just a possibility. They don't know everything. I reckon it was caused by that bash from the table. If you find a lump obviously we'll have to get it sorted, and we'll face that if we have to. But please don't go terrifying yourself about things that aren't there.'

I knew that was true, but at times I just could not stop crying. I felt I was going to be the ruin of our family. We had all been so happy, so fortunate that I had survived the lymphoma. Not a day had gone by since I had finished the steroid treatment that I did not think about cancer and wonder if it would come back. Now, here I was almost actively seeking it. How could I endanger Ger and the kids like this? How could I do something that might take me away from them for ever? How on earth was I going to survive the next eight months of this? It couldn't be good for the baby if the mother was a nervous wreck – I had read that the adrenalin flooding my system from anxiety and stress could cross the placenta. I willed myself to calm down.

Appointments had been made for me at the same hospital where I had been treated for the lymphoma. I was to go for regular check-ups with the obstetrician, and after each one I was booked in with my oncologist. The twelve-week appointment was looming – the first time I had been back in the hospital since dropping the bombshell.

'Ger, can you come with me to the hospital next week? I have an appointment to check the baby, then I need to see your man again.' I couldn't say his name, I refused to think I might become a cancer patient again.

It seemed odd to be going to a different department, turning down unfamiliar corridors, but once we were through the heavy swing doors of the gynaecology and obstetrics department we might just as well have been in a different world altogether. There was the sound of lively chatter, and parenting magazines and children's toys filled the waiting areas. Everyone seemed cheerful, healthy, comparing bumps and due dates. The receptionist was smiling. It struck me forcefully: pregnancy wasn't a disease, it was a state of positive health in which a woman's body tends towards strength and vitality. We sat down next to a red-faced young woman who looked as if she might give birth any moment. Ger raised a mild eyebrow.

'Hello,' she breathed. 'I was due six days ago and I'm here to find out if I need to be induced.' We chatted for a bit, and I explained I was here for my twelve-week scan. While we were waiting, one of the nurses took me aside for the standard urine test, blood test and blood-pressure check. I returned to find her still firing questions at Ger.

'Is this your first baby?' she asked me. 'How have you been feeling?' For once I was lost for words, and I looked over at Ger for help. Luckily her name was called at that moment.

'I don't feel like a normal pregnant person,' I whispered to Ger.

'You're not. You're my wife,' he rejoined.

The obstetrician was a jolly grey-haired woman in her fifties. She immediately put us at our ease as she asked all the usual questions about my other pregnancies, dates, blood group, family history and so on. She then examined me, gently pressing my abdomen to check the position of the top of the womb. Then she frowned slightly.

'Is everything all right?' I asked. I knew that, as a forty-year-old, I already stood a greater risk of something going wrong with the pregnancy – let alone the other risks we knew about.

'Mrs Bohan, I know your history. I can quite understand how you are feeling – this must be a terribly worrying time for you both. However, I am going to assume that everything is going to be fine. To me you are just another pregnant woman. Right, let's have a look at this baby then.' She switched on the screen.

I have always loved the way an ultrasound scan gives you a brief window on the secret life within you. That day Ger and I watched the mass of swirls on the screen and tried to decipher the vague outline of a tiny form. The obstetrician pointed out the head, spine and feet. I could see it throbbing.

'There's the heartbeat!' she exclaimed. 'And, looking at these measurements, your baby seems absolutely fine.' She printed out a floppy black and white print for me to take. I felt an absurd rush of love for this fuzzy blob, and was unable to speak for a few moments.

'I would like to see you every month from now on until you are six months pregnant, after which we can relax a little more. If you have any questions or problems, or anything unusual crops up, give me a call. In the meantime, do try and enjoy your pregnancy. You're going to be fine.' She ushered us out of her consulting room and we made our way over to the receptionist to sort out the next few appointments.

Gerard looked at his watch. 'We're just in time for the oncologist.' My excitement at having seen our baby on the scan suddenly evaporated, and we walked slowly down the corridor full of dread. Now I had seen it on the screen I wanted to protect it all the more. If the cancer had come back I made up my mind to refuse any treatment until it was born. Ger's face was grim. I decided not to tell him what I was thinking.

'Hello, Bernadette,' said the oncologist. We were on first-name terms. 'You know the routine.' I certainly did. In a few moments I was lying on the familiar couch, praying silently as he checked my entire body. Ger was sitting biting his lip. It was very quiet.

'You're fine,' the oncologist said eventually. 'Everything looks grand: I can't find any sign that the cancer is presenting. You can get dressed.'

It had been raining that morning but it started to clear as we drove back to Malahide, where we lived. The roads were wet and the fields we passed all had a clean, just-washed look. We were both enormously relieved that I was – so far – doing well, but I felt a growing sense of more than relief. Suddenly I felt clear headed and positive. I decided to follow the obstetrician's advice and enjoy my pregnancy. I wasn't going to get anywhere by worrying – it wasn't going to help me, it wasn't going to help my family and it certainly would not help the baby. It was time to stop fighting it and trust that God would show me the way.

That evening we told Sarah I was expecting. 'Oh, Mammy! I'm going to be a big sister! That's so exciting!' she yelled with glee and rushed outside to tell Richard who was as usual kicking a ball around the back garden. As we listened to their animated chattering ('It's going to be a boy'; 'No it's not, it's going to be a girl!') we got caught up in their delight.

'I really believe this is going to be fine,' I stated confidently. 'Today I have made a conscious decision not to worry any more. This baby is a gift from God and I am determined to enjoy my pregnancy, not live in fear every minute.'

'I'll drink to that,' said Gerard happily, uncorking a bottle. We joined the children in the garden, and from that moment on I refused to allow myself to be afraid. Every time the worry popped into my mind, as it did from time to time, I deliberately shut it down.

I went on to have an uneventful pregnancy. I grew bigger with each passing month, and grew too in my sense of joy and fulfil-ment. I went to the hospital each month for the double whammy of obstetrician/oncologist, and although I never got used to the stark contrast between the light and hope of one department and the fear and coldness of the other, I kept telling myself that God was looking after me and this was all part of His plan.

It was thrilling for me to feel the baby's first squirming, wrig-gling movements around the eighteenth week, and I'll never for-get taking both the children to the twenty-week scan. The look on their faces when they saw the cloudy outline of their new brother or sister and listened to the soft whooshing of the blood flow will stay with me for ever. The obstetrician spent a long time pointing out the fingers and toes, and we could even make out the profile of the face.

'It's waving at us,' giggled Sarah, as the baby moved slightly at the pressure from the scanning wand.

'That's my brother,' said Richard.

'I'm convinced it's a boy,' I said conversationally to the obstetrician. She gave me an old-fashioned look, from which I guessed that Richard wouldn't be getting his footballer after all. I would have to tell him before the birth. In fact I broke it to him later. 'That's OK, Mum,' he said. 'Girls can play football too.'

I became calmer and more serene in the final months, practising yoga and meditation techniques that seemed to give me inner strength and helped make me more accepting of anything that was to happen. The deep breathing gave me time to think and be myself. This was going to be my last baby, I knew that for certain. She would be like me, the youngest of the family. I remember having vivid dreams at the end of my pregnancy, particularly about my own childhood. Leafing through some old photo albums of Richard and Sarah as young children I remembered how sweet they had been to each other in those days, and I longed for the day when we would have another little one amongst us.

Everything I did at that stage was focussed on the coming birth. My world became smaller and quieter. I took down Richard's cradle from the attic, which I had been keeping for his children, and washed and ironed the tiny sheets and cellular blankets. With it I found two little sleepsuits of his that I couldn't part with when I had my big clear-out after my miscarriage. I would have to buy some more, I realized, and Sarah would just love to come shopping with me. 'It will be like having a real live doll,' I promised her.

'I'm astonished,' said my oncologist one afternoon late into my pregnancy, just after another routine check with the obstetrician. I was due to give birth in a month's time. 'You have confounded my expectations – you are as healthy a patient as I have ever seen. Well done.' That was praise indeed from him.

'What are we going to call the baby?' asked Sarah one morning, and we all laughed to think we hadn't got any names decided on, even though my due date was coming up fast. The children drew up a list of names, and Ger and I scanned baby-name books for inspiration. None of us could agree on any names we liked, until one evening when we were sitting watching the credits roll up after a film. 'Julie,' I read. 'That's nice.' Everyone nodded. So Julie it was.

Because of my age, the doctor decided to induce me six days early, so unlike the other children who had arrived at very unsociable hours, Julie's birth was very civilized. We left Sarah and Richard with Ger's mother and 'checked in' at the hospital at 8am. They broke my waters, and having been told things would take some hours to get moving, Ger nipped off to a meeting. When he returned a few hours later we walked around a little, hoping that would speed the process up. At midday we rang the kids to let them know nothing had happened yet. Finally, Julie was born at 5.20 that afternoon. The midwife handed me a mewling bundle.

'She looks Chinese!' I gasped.

'She'd better not be or there'll be a steward's enquiry,' said Ger.

I looked down at my tiny newborn baby girl who was already staring at me with dark eyes. 'Hello, Julie,' I murmured. 'I'm your Mummy. I've been waiting to meet you for ages!' She looked strong – she would be a fighter, like me. I knew she was going to be fine.

That evening the kids turned up with their Granny, Anne. Sarah was chatting away about a gift someone had sent for Julie, but Richard just stared at her silently, totally overwhelmed. I could see this was the most amazing thing that had ever happened to him, and little did he know then how much she would come to mean to him. Baby Julie was and is the joy of all our lives. To anyone else of course she is just a normal kid, but to us she is a little miracle. Richard and Sarah now look after her like parents, watching out for her and caring for her. On the day she was born I thought I would burst with happiness, but each day of her life she has made me even happier. Julie has filled a part of me that I thought I had lost.

So it wasn't poor Bernadette after all. It was blessed, lucky Bernadette. I had been given my longed-for third child: my family was complete, my world was whole and the future looked wonderful.

Chapter Eleven

Stress

People always ask me if stress causes cancer. There is so much written these days about stress, stress hormones, stressful life events, and all the different ways of dealing with stress. I'm not a medical person so I couldn't really say if stress actually causes cancer, but I do know this much. When you are stressed you stop looking after yourself properly. You miss meals, you forget to drink enough water, you don't sleep properly, you have no time to exercise, you may keep yourself going with sugary snacks, alcohol and cigarettes, perhaps even drugs. And when you stop looking after yourself you are looking for trouble.

We are jumping five years on in my story. Richard was seventeen, Sarah was fifteen and Julie was five, so life was busy as it is for any parent with two children in secondary school and one starting junior school – not to mention George, our boisterous Labrador. I was always on the go, with very little time for myself, but that was the life I had chosen, and it was very much what I wanted. I never forgot that I had been given the gift of more time with them, the chance to see them grow up, and I thanked God every day for this. Of course it was exhausting and difficult at times, but so rewarding to watch them develop and change and to be able to relate to them on different levels. They are all so different but all such gorgeous kids, and really give me very little trouble. Of course the rascals now get up to all the usual teenage carry-on – staying out late, playing loud music, random sulks. But one of the things I appreciate the most is that I feel they talk to me – they really open up about what is upsetting them and what they are excited about. When I was growing up I had secrets from my parents, and they had secrets from me. Ger and I have tried very hard to be open and honest with our children so that they not only are straight and honest with us, but trust us to be straight with them.

I felt fortunate to have such easy-going kids, and I could not imagine how women with more complicated lives coped. Yet despite this, and despite being fairly health-conscious even in those days, I tended to grab food on the run and simply did not spend much time taking care of myself. The kids came first, no question, and my needs were always the last on the list. Like many mothers I was cook, chauffeur, nurse, homework-supervisor, cleaner, confidante and sergeant-major all rolled into one. I also made their clothes and did the same for friends, which kept me awake into the small hours. When I look back at this period now, I think it was far more stressful than I realized. I had no idea what problems I might be storing up for myself.

Then two things happened that took me way off the stress scale.

Like many women in their forties I was also partly responsible for my ageing mother, who at this stage was suffering from mild dementia but was adamant she wanted to stay in her own home. To facilitate this, my sister Aquinas – who lived close to her – went to see her every day. My brother Frank sometimes stopped for the night with her, and I would drive thirty miles each week to visit her. Then one day the phone rang. It was Aquinas.

'It's Mum. She's had a stroke.'

I suppose when your parent is old you expect to hear news like this all the time, but nevertheless it was a shock.

'Jesus, Aquinas, how bad is it?'

'It's only mild, they say, but she's in hospital. I can't cope with her any more on my own – I'm going to need help from the rest of you.'

Poor Aquinas was worn ragged with all the caring she did, and I knew she needed help, so I drove up to the hospital and back every second day. It wasn't easy to arrange all this, but by this time Richard and Sarah were old enough to babysit Julie if I wasn't around. 'I'm sorry, you two,' I'd say. 'You're on duty again this afternoon. I need to go and visit Granny.'

Fortunately my mother recovered, but was unable to live alone after this. It was decided that she would move in with Aquinas. Again, in order to help my sister, I offered to have her to stay with me for the first few days, so I drove her back to our house on the Friday night. As I was installing her in the spare room, Sarah appeared.

'I've got a headache, Mum.'

'Have you? Have a little rest. I expect you'll feel better later. Did you have a tough day at school?'

'Yeah, I suppose.'

The next day I left Mum in Richard's care while I went shopping for some things she needed. Sarah had a Saturday job in the local newsagent's and I popped in to say hello.

'Ooh, my cheek feels numb,' she commented, rubbing her face. 'And so does my arm.'

'Numb? What do you think caused that?' I asked, a little absent-mindedly, as I checked over my shopping list.

'I don't know. It's like when you have been to the dentist.'

Not another of Sarah's aches and pains, I sighed to myself. If it wasn't one thing, it was another: I couldn't keep up with these small but rather regular teenage problems, and I usually found they disappeared in time if I ignored them.

'I expect you'll feel better later. See you this evening – make sure you're home in time for dinner.'

Ger was away on business and I had a hard time dealing with everything that weekend. Nothing I did for my mother was quite right, and I was trying my best to keep an even temper.

Julie was making a racket on her recorder, Richard was having trouble with his Geography coursework, and Sarah was still complaining of a headache.

On Monday after school she said it was worse. 'Perhaps you're brewing up 'flu or something,' I suggested. 'Why don't you lie on the couch and have a rest?' That way, I thought, she'd be one fewer problem for me to deal with.

On Tuesday she took the day off school. I took my mother back to Aquinas, then drove straight to the airport to fetch Ger. When we got back, there was Sarah, looking pale and tired.

'I don't think I can bear this headache much longer.' This was one problem that clearly was not going to go away. Suddenly I was worried.

'Right. Sit down and tell me exactly how you feel.'

'Both my cheeks are numb, and I have a splitting headache.' A small worm of fear crept into my mind. Numbness. A headache that doesn't go.

'OK, Sarah, get in the car. I'm taking you to hospital.' I grabbed her coat, bundled her into the car and rushed to Casualty. They immediately gave her a brain scan.

A brain scan? Sweet Jesus what have I done? The poor lassie has been trying to tell me something for days now and I have been ignoring her! I felt like the worst mother in the entire universe.

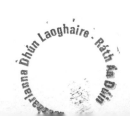

'God, I'm sorry Sarah. I should have brought you here days ago.'

'It's OK, Mum. Don't worry.' Very gently, I took her into the waiting area and sat down with my arms around her. We sat like that for a very long time, and she eventually fell asleep with her head on my lap. All sorts of unimaginable horrors were running through my mind as I drifted in and out of sleep, trying to stay alert for Sarah but achingly tired, praying all the while to God that she was going to be all right. While she slept I rang Ger to let him know what was happening. He came in around four in the morning to relieve me.

'You go home, Bernie. You need to get some sleep.'

'Sleep? There's no way I'll be able to sleep until I know what's up with Sarah.'

We waited together for the results of the scan to come and for a doctor to tell us what was wrong. Finally a nurse appeared.

'I can't tell you anything yet, but we are definitely admitting her.' She took us up to a ward, and Sarah was laid in a curtained-off bed. We tried not to jump to any conclusions, but I knew from Ger's face that his thoughts were as dark as mine. We hung around waiting, waiting, waiting. When Sarah woke up I told her I would pop home, have a wash and collect her nightclothes. 'OK, Mum. Don't be long.'

I drove like a madwoman, praying out loud, only just able to see the road through my hot tears. *Dear God, please don't do this to her.*

Don't let her suffer, she's only a kid.

I got home just after breakfast. Julie, who was just learning to write, was painstakingly making a little Get Well card for Sarah. Richard was clearing away breakfast.

'How is she, Mum?' he asked. I knew he was dreadfully worried. Only the previous day Richard and Sarah had been hurling insults at each other. Now, when the chips were down, I saw how deeply he cared for her.

'We don't know yet, they've done some tests and will be keeping her in for a bit. Could you take Julie to school for me?' Julie ran over with her card, which was sticky with glue and sequins.

'Can't I come with you now so I can give it to Sarah?'

'Well, why don't we let it dry first? You have a lovely day at school, then perhaps we'll take it to her later if she's still in hospital.'

I grabbed a few things for Sarah, kissed them both goodbye, and rushed out of the house. When I got back to Sarah she told me the surgeon had already done his rounds. Shit, I'd missed him. Ger had gone to work to cancel his arrangements for the day.

'Mum, he said I have a cyst on my brain.' She said it in a matter-of-fact voice but her eyes were scared.

'What?' I almost screamed. What did that mean, and what were they doing giving this news to a fifteen-year-old on her own?

'It's not serious, really – it's OK. They are going to monitor me.'

'That's grand. I'll just see if I can find the doctor.' I couldn't help it, my eyes filled with tears, and I turned so Sarah would not see.

The neurosurgeon, when I had tracked him down, was not quite as positive with me as he had been with Sarah. He told me it was definitely a lump, but he did not know exactly what it was. She would need to stay in for more tests.

Later, in the ward, Sarah lay on the metal bed surrounded by three senior surgeons. The big guns. They planned a series of tests for her – CT scans, MRI scans and others I had never heard of. One of the machines broke down, so the waiting was more drawn-out than it should have been. In all, she was in hospital for nine days, and I was by her side as much as I could. I swear to God there is nothing in this world worse than having a sick child. Every protective instinct in your body is focussed on making them better, on taking care of them as you have from the moment they were conceived, but when they are in hospital your power to do this is taken away from you. All your love, your hopes, your prayers – all contract into this one hospital room, this one small bed. I remembered children I had met in the other hospital where I had been treated for the lymphoma – children with white faces and dull eyes. I remembered how even if they were smiling, playing with toys or doing something apparently normal, they seemed marked out as different, tragic. I wondered if any of them were still living. Now I understood how their parents felt, why they seemed to wander around the corridors as if sleep-walking. Why they showered their children with gifts and sweets. And I wondered if there was a cancer 'gene' I had passed on to my child. Was this a brain tumour?

The only thing I knew I definitely could do was pray, so I prayed then like never before. In the days of waiting, it made me feel as if I was able to do something small for her. And I made a desperate bargain: *Take me, God. Don't take Sarah. Make her well and do what you want to me. I can handle it. I know I can cope, I've done it before. She's too young for this. If someone has to suffer let it be me. Take me in exchange for her. Take me.*

Ger dropped in on his way to work each morning, and after I had taken Julie to school I went and sat by her bedside all day. Later in the day I would pick Julie up again, then the both of us would go and chat with her until it was time for Julie to go home to bed. It broke my heart to see her lying there so scared, waiting for yet another test, but we did our utmost to keep her spirits up. Somehow word spread around the village, neighbours and friends called in non-stop to see how she was doing, and it seemed to me as if every kid in Malahide came to visit her in the ward. She even celebrated her sixteenth birthday there, with helium balloons, two cakes and more presents than she had ever received. I realized all her friends thought she was dying.

I was worried that having a party in the hospital would disturb the older patients, but they were so accepting.

'No, love, let her be. She's life in the ward. It does us good to see her.' They were more than accepting. These thin, wasted souls yearned for the invigorating energy of young people. They loved

Sarah, I could see. And she had them wrapped around her little finger.

Happily, Sarah's headaches gradually disappeared, and she presented no new signs. Then finally we were given the results of all the tests.

'Mrs Bohan, your daughter has an arachnoid cyst on the left anterior wall of her brain. It is possibly left over from the embryonic stage, but in any event because of the location we have decided not to remove it – unless in the future she becomes severely affected by it.'

'Oh, thank you so much!' I shook the hand of the neurosurgeon who gave us the news. 'That's wonderful news.' Sarah was beaming.

'Do you need to see her back again for check-ups or anything?'

'Yes, we'll need to see her every four months or so, and of course you should come in immediately if there are any problems.'

Naturally I was overwhelmed with relief, but at the same time knew this would now be a constant worry: I would always be on the look out for new signs of trouble, and I would certainly never ignore any of her headaches again.

'WELLCOM HOM SARAH!!!' read the banner on our front door. Julie was thrilled to have her big sister back, and that night we had a little celebration at home.

'Mum, Dad, can I have another birthday party now I'm back home?' she asked. 'That wasn't really a proper party in the hospital.'

'Of course you can,' we smiled, knowing that at that moment we would have given her the sun, the moon and the stars.

As I sank into bed that night I thanked God fervently for answering my prayers and keeping her safe and well.

One month later I discovered a lump in my own breast.

Chapter Twelve

Every Woman's Nightmare

'It can't be,' I said to myself as I felt under my arm for the hundredth time. It was – I had to admit – a definite lump, around two centimetres in diameter. Gerard was at work and the children were at school – there was no one to ask, no one to tell me I was imagining it, no one to make me feel normal. There it was again – hardish, rather sore. Nasty lumps aren't meant to be sore, but my lymphoma had been sore so what did that prove? I sat on the bed to think. I had been cancer-free for twelve years, and after five years you are considered 'cured', so it seemed unlikely that this was a tumour. (I did not know then that I had a far greater chance of developing cancer again than someone who had never had cancer.) I thought of the million times I had checked myself over the past twelve years – usually in the bath or shower, when I was alone with myself. I was assiduous – I would check not just my breasts and groin but every single part of me. When you have had cancer you live with it and the possibility of its return every day of your life. Yet I was shocked at finding this lump. I felt it again and frowned. Perhaps I had pulled a muscle at the gym. Perhaps it was part of the lumpiness I often felt before a period. Whatever it was, I did not like it.

'Ger, would you come up here?' I called, as soon as I heard his key in the door that evening. The children were asleep and he was late home. I'd thought of nothing else all afternoon.

'What is it?' he asked, sensing the urgency in my voice.

'I've found a lump ...' he was by my side in a trice, 'here.' He felt it, and nodded.

'Hmm. I see what you mean. Look, of course you're worried, anyone would be, with your history,' he tried to reassure me. 'But I'm sure it's nothing – you couldn't be unlucky enough to get hit a second time. Put it out of your mind until you can get it checked out.'

'I'll wait until my period comes to see if it goes away – it might just be the time of the month.'

'OK, but don't mess around, Bernie. Don't wait too long.'

A few days later I saw my GP, who got on the phone instantly. He discovered that my usual oncologist was on holiday at that time, so he booked me in for an appointment with another specialist.

This doctor was young and fresh-faced. He smiled nervously as he examined me. I ought to be the nervous one, I thought.

'I think I'll just do a needle biopsy,' he said. 'It's a simple pro-cedure in which I remove a few cells from the lump and send them off to the lab for analysis.' I was surprised that he could do it then and there, but pleased that the first step was being taken this quickly. I felt a deep stab of pain as the needle went in – after all the injections and tests I had had before, this one felt particularly sore, perhaps because the needle was going into one of the softest, most personal parts of my body. I shut my eyes and pretended I wasn't there. As he transferred the contents of the syringe to a slide he carried on talking.

'The results of a test like this aren't always conclusive, so don't be surprised if we call you back for a further test, what we call a core biopsy.'

'Should I be worried? I'm about to go on holiday for two weeks.'

'Oh no, we won't get the results until next Tuesday anyway, and if we need to book you in for another test that can wait until your return. Are you going somewhere nice?'

I explained that we were going to Fuerte Ventura, in the Canaries. We hadn't had a holiday for some time and although Richard couldn't come with us – he was going off to Greece with his friends later in August – the girls were really excited. He asked me how old the children were, and then he told me that he had been two years ago with his girlfriend and had had a wonderful time surfing – the waves were superb.

'I don't expect I'll be doing much of that! In fact I don't know how I'm going to relax at all with this hanging over me.'

'Try and put it out of your mind and give us a call when you get back. Have a lovely holiday – and don't spend it worrying.'

Yet it was with a heavy heart that I set off on that year's family holiday. Not that I was normally the superstitious kind, but there did seem to be an awful parallel with that other holiday twelve years ago when we discovered the first lump. It was June again, we were off to the Canary Islands again, and Julie was now just about the same age as Sarah had been then. Surely, surely, this could not be happening all over again?

Sensible, practical Gerard wouldn't hear of this '*déjà vu*' talk – and he did his best to keep up all our spirits that fortnight.

He couldn't stop me from phoning the hospital, though, on the Tuesday I knew the test results would be in. I made the call from a café near our beach, and it was a bad line. It took the hospital some time to put me through to the doctor, and I could barely hear his voice.

'Mrs Bohan? Yes, we have your results here – but as I predicted we are going to have to get you back in again for the core biopsy.' I froze. What did this mean? The pips went and I fumbled in my shorts' pocket for more coins, dropping some on the floor in my hurry.

'Are you still there?' he was shouting, but faint.

'What is it? Is it the cancer back?' I made myself say the words.

'Look, it is standard practice; it doesn't mean there is anything sinister there. We'll see you at the end of the month. Don't worry.' I put the phone down: I was running out of coins and he wasn't going to tell me what I wanted to hear. Making my way slowly back to where the others were waiting on the beach, I wondered what to tell them. I desperately needed to talk about this, but I didn't want to ruin their holiday. I didn't want to ruin mine either – perhaps it was just a routine test, after all. Spotting them in the distance I increased my pace and jogged off to join them.

When I reached them, panting, Gerard raised his eyebrows as if to say, 'Well?'

I shrugged my shoulders and said simply: 'I have to go back.' He wrapped me in his arms right there, in the middle of the beach, and said, 'It doesn't mean anything – yet. Try not to let it get to you. Whatever happens, we're all together and we all love you.'

Later that day I was lying on a beach towel while Sarah put sun cream on my back. She and I were good companions that holiday – Julie and Ger were always off rushing in and out of the waves and building castles with great moats for the sea to swallow. Julie was an active, happy little girl and adored playing games with her Dad. Sarah was sixteen and just entering that stage when girls turn into women and start to gain at least a veneer of understanding of how the adult world works. She loved hearing stories from my childhood, about her aunts and uncles, and about how I met Gerard. She was just beginning to go out with boys herself and was fascinated by other people's relationships, so in a way it was a bit like having a girlfriend on holiday with me.

But that afternoon I could think of nothing but the lump, and my conversation with the doctor, and what might follow a core biopsy. I was loath to burden Sarah with too much knowledge, but perhaps there was a way I could prepare her gently.

'Sarah, pet, do you have any memory of when I was sick all those years ago?'

'Yes, sort of. I remember you couldn't walk very well and you got fat. I know you had cancer of the something. But you took some tablets and got well again, didn't you?'

'I did, yes. But I have another lump now and I'm worried. I don't know what I'll do if the cancer has returned.'

She turned her big green eyes on me, and they were full of love and understanding. 'Don't worry, Mum, everything will be all right. Really it will.' She sounded so grown-up, so confident, so reassuring. I desperately wanted to believe her.

As it turned out, everything was far from all right.

On our return from the Canaries I was called in for a mammogram – apparently they wanted to explore every avenue before my oncologist returned. Gerard was busy that day and could not get out of work, so I asked my friend Grace to come with me. Grace is one of my best friends and was a fantastic support during the months ahead – whatever was happening she and I always managed to have a good bit of craic together. Having a mammogram is an extraordinary experience, quite unlike a normal X-ray where you lie prone on a table. Standing next to the machine, I had to lean forward and put as much of my breast as I could onto a glass plate, and it was then squashed as flat as a pancake by another hard plate. I have small breasts and this was not an easy manoeuvre.

'The compression may cause some discomfort,' advised the radiographer as she saw me wince. Discomfort, I thought, that weasel word again.

'It is important for us to obtain maximum compression in order to achieve good resolution on the mammograms. Otherwise we may miss small lesions.' Fair enough, I grimaced, but hurry up. Was I imagining it, or was the breast with the lump sorer than the other one?

The X-ray pictures were developed immediately and were examined by the radiographer. As I got dressed I looked at the pictures on the screen. I could make out a distinct lump but it did not seem to be connected to anything – perhaps it was just a cyst.

'What do you think?' I asked her.

'Oh, I only take the pictures. You'll have to talk to your doctor about what they mean. My job is to make sure they're not blurred. I'll pass them along to the radiologist who will send a report to your surgeon. I expect you'll hear from him with the results in a few days.'

I was making the children their breakfast a few days later when the phone rang. It was my oncologist's secretary. He was still on holiday but his office was in charge of my notes.

'Hello, Claire,' I said, instantly on my guard. 'What's the news?'

'We'd like you to go to the public hospital this morning for the results of your mammogram and to have the core biopsy.'

'Why do I need to go to that hospital? Can't I wait until he is back from holiday?'

'Well, there's no need to keep you waiting for him. I'm sure you want to get the results as soon as possible.' She was giving nothing away, but I was heartened by her positive, sunny tone.

There was no time to organize a babysitter for Julie that morning – but I called Gerard and thankfully he was able to come with us to the hospital and had arranged to keep the rest of the day free. We agreed to meet outside, and I was pleased to see him arrive early despite the Dublin traffic. As we walked into the hospital Ger asked me how I was feeling.

'Fine, actually. I think they have been extra-careful with me because of my history. Having a core biopsy is routine, and I couldn't see anything suspicious on the X-ray. Maybe I'm wrong, but Claire sounded quite jolly this morning – I know her so well I'm sure I would have picked up on any problems.' Julie was running ahead down the corridor, looking into all the open doors. We were out of breath when we eventually reached the unfamiliar waiting room.

'Let's have a barbecue tonight,' said Ger after we had announced ourselves to the receptionist.

'Yes, let's do that. We'll shop at Superquinn on the way back.'

'OK, and can we stop off at the garden centre? I'd like to get some plants and start on the far left corner in the garden. And I need some bits at the hardware shop.' We chatted for a while about our other plans for the day – it was unusual for us to have a whole day together and it would be good to get all the various little household jobs done.

'I wish they'd hurry up. I want to get on,' grumbled Gerard after nearly an hour. 'Look at all these other people waiting.' At least Julie was unconcerned about the wait, watching the tropical fish in a tank in the corner of the room.

Finally my name was called. I left Gerard with Julie and went in alone. It was a surgeon I didn't recognize, with a nurse behind him fiddling with some needles and stuff. I sat down and looked at him expectantly. He was shuffling his papers.

'Mrs Bohan, from the tests we have done so far I can make a conclusive diagnosis.' He paused. I noticed he did not meet my eyes – a classic warning sign. 'There is no easy way to say this. You have breast cancer.' My heart stopped. They must have made a mistake.

'Are you sure? Have you mixed up the tests? Can I see the notes?'

'I'm afraid I am sure. These are definitely your results. I am in no doubt, looking at the needle biopsy results and the mammogram. I'm sorry.'

I did not know what to say. I couldn't believe it, simply could not take the information in. I had had cancer once before, and now I was being told I had it again. No! I screamed inside. It can't be happening again. To get this news once was bad, but twice! Sweet Jesus, this was too cruel for words. I suddenly felt cold, and started to shiver all over. The nurse handed me a blanket and tucked it around me.

'Will I get your husband for you?' she asked kindly.

'No, he's with my little girl. She's only five – we can't leave her on her own.' I turned to the surgeon and tried to gather my thoughts. 'What happens next?'

'Well, er, the breast will come off, along with the lymph glands, after which you will have radiation and chemo. Then we may remove some of the muscle from your back to reconstruct the breast. You won't have a nipple.' I wasn't taking this in. It sound-ed horrendous, drastic. I couldn't understand why my back would be involved – it was bad enough taking my breast, but to cut into my back? A terrible image of a carved-out back and a sliced-off breast flashed through my mind. This couldn't be happening. This on top of the terrible destruction sure to be wreaked by the cancer.

I pulled my top back on and walked outside. I was having trouble breathing. Ger told me afterwards he knew something was very wrong as soon as he saw me – I was deathly pale. Standing against a door, I motioned to him to come over. Julie was playing happily on the floor with some toys. The door I was leaning against swung open and I almost fell over. It was the gents' toilets. Ger grabbed hold of me. I shook my head in despair.

'It's back.' I blurted out. 'The cancer is back.'

His reaction was instant. He just held me, and didn't let go for a long time.

'We'll get through this. We'll handle it, we'll be all right,' he kept saying, as much to convince himself, I thought after, as to reassure me. I tried to tell him about the chemotherapy and the radiotherapy and the terrifying operation and then there was the nurse again, telling me gently it was time to go in for the core biopsy.

'Ger, it might be better for Julie not to be with us this afternoon – can you call your mother and get her to take care of her?' He nodded encouragingly to me as I went back into the surgeon's consulting room.

The core biopsy, I was told, was the final test that would confirm beyond doubt that the cancer had indeed returned. My mind was such a blur that day, but I'll never forget the sight of the unnaturally long needle which he plunged into my breast again and again from different angles to extract tissue for examination. I can't remember if he used an anaesthetic, but in my state of shock I hardly felt it.

'I've called Mum,' said Gerard when I came out again, 'I had to give her the news, but she's in such a state we can't possibly leave Julie with her. She's worse than we are – there's no way she'd be able to hold it together. Julie would definitely know something was wrong.'

This hospital was right next door to my original hospital, and I had been told I'd have to go and make an appointment to see my oncologist. Leaving Julie and Gerard outside his office, I went to find Claire. She looked at me when I went in, and when she saw my face such a look of sympathy crossed hers. She knew everything. I just stood there and wept. She is not a demonstrative woman, but she put her arm round my shoulders in a gesture that, for her, spoke volumes. I made the appointment, dried my eyes and walked out – putting a brave face on things for my little Julie's sake. And I had to hold it together for the rest of the day – it was a Friday and Julie usually stayed up late for a special supper with us. We so badly wanted to be by ourselves, but we also did not want to give any hint that anything out of the ordinary was happening.

We were driving home from the hospital, with Julie sitting quietly in the car. I wondered if she had picked up our distress and looked nervously over at her. Suddenly Ger's mobile rang. It was Sarah. My God, Sarah! We'd have to tell her.

'Dad, have you seen the doctor? What did he say? What's wrong with Mum?' Sarah fired a volley of questions at him while he was driving. I looked at him, indicating Julie with a jerk of my head, hoping he wouldn't let anything slip. I needn't have worried. He was monosyllabic in his answers to her, 'Yes … no … tell you later … yeah … it's back … OK.'

Poor Sarah, she had vomited at work that day – she had literally been worried sick about me. Her colleagues had laughed at her, assuming she was hung over after a big night out. She had a holiday job in one of Gerard's shops, and she had promised him not to say anything about my tests. He was always concerned to keep his private life separate from his professional life – and never gave anything away. After all, he reasoned, I don't want to give anyone any reason to suspect that – in any confrontational situation – I may be thought to be bringing my personal problems into work. It was not that he was ashamed, he just needed to keep work and home separate. There would be a time to tell people, but it certainly was not now.

Gerard put the phone down. 'She took it OK, don't worry. She said she'd be all right to carry on at work until the end of the day and she'd see us later.'

It seemed like a lifetime ago that we had been chatting about what we would do that day. And, like automata, we did every-thing we'd planned: we bought the plants, we did the grocery shopping, Gerard cut the grass, we put up some shelves and he fixed a wobbly gate. We even cooked a lunchtime barbecue with Julie, letting her throw the sausages on the top and help mix up the spicy sauce. All this we did in a kind of daze, not talking about it because of Julie, holding our shattering news inside our-selves, and watching other people carrying out their business, completely unaware of the turmoil we were feeling.

They were normal; we were different – and things would never be the same again.

Chapter Thirteen

Breaking the News

N o one knows how they are going to react at times like this. Some people need to be alone; others need to be with a crowd of people. Some people want to discuss the diagnosis, their fears and the treatment with everyone they meet; others withdraw into themselves and are unwilling to discuss anything at all. For me, it was something of a blessing that my friend Maria, who lived in Italy, was staying with us that weekend.

Maria is a lively, boisterous woman and was the breath of fresh air and normality we needed. We told her the news when she returned from a shopping trip late that afternoon, and she sat down suddenly, saying simply, 'Oh my God, no.' Within moments she had pulled herself together and grabbed Julie's hand, muttering something about having lots of good games to play in the garden. I took refuge in the kitchen to prepare the evening meal, and watched them from the window playing Grandmother's Footsteps and Hide and Seek. I felt glad she was there. Gerard opened a bottle of wine and handed me a glass. It was the first drink I'd had since getting the news, and as the alcohol warmed the back of my throat I realized how much I needed to relax. I was wound as tightly as a spring.

Richard was due back at any moment from his holiday job in the record shop at the airport. Unlike Sarah, he had not called to find out what happened at the hospital, but I knew it would have been on his mind all day. I felt a sudden pang for my only son. How on earth was I going to drop this bombshell on him? He was eighteen, and had just finished his Leaving Certificate. This news was going to be a crushing blow.

'Ger, I don't know how I'm going to tell Richard. I just don't think I can do it without breaking down. I'm trying really hard to keep it together.'

'I know, I know. Don't worry, I'll tell him,' Ger reassured me.

As soon as he came through the door Richard looked at me, questioning. I hugged him hello, then Ger beckoned him into the lounge and sat down on the couch with him. I could just hear Gerard's voice.

'Richard, Mum had some bad news today. The cancer is back. She will need an operation, chemotherapy and all the rest.' I couldn't hear Richard's reply, then a few minutes later the door slammed shut and Richard raced upstairs two at a time. I didn't follow him – I knew he needed to be by himself. I would talk to him later.

Normally family meals in our house are rowdy affairs, with Sarah and Richard squabbling, the two of us laughing and chatting, Julie entertaining us with her random thoughts, the clatter of plates and clinking of glasses. But that evening we were all

absorbed in our own thoughts. Ger and I were uncharacteristi-
cally quiet, and throughout dinner Richard sat and watched me
with eyes that could have bored holes in me. He did not take his
gaze off me all evening – while I was serving, while I was eating.
He hardly touched his meal and wouldn't talk about the holiday
he was planning to take with some friends. I kept seeing him
struggling to compose himself, taking deep breaths as if he was
trying to stop himself keeling over. I knew that by staring at me
he was trying to read my mind, wordlessly begging for reassurance that I was all right. Maria, on the other hand, rose to the
occasion tremendously and yakked on about anything and everything, over-compensating for our silence and keeping us all
going until the meal was over. Sarah was amazing, too, and she
chipped in with news about the village, about her friends, about
what she was doing. Yet the atmosphere was heavy with the one
big subject none of us could discuss because Julie was with us. As
soon as dinner was over Sarah asked if she could go out with
her friends.

'Of course you can – what time will you be back?'

'Around twelve. You go to bed, Mum, if you're tired. Don't wait
up.' I knew what she was doing, and I understood. My Sarah, at
sixteen, would have stayed out half the night, given the chance.
Tonight it did not seem so important to check up on her, and I
knew she knew we had enough going on without having to worry
about her staying out too late.

After clearing up I went upstairs to get Julie's pyjamas. Maria
was out on the patio drinking wine and chatting to Ger – their

last chance to talk before she returned to Italy the next day. Julie was playing happily with her dolls next to them. I glanced into Richard's room as I passed. He had his back to me, but I could see he was fiddling with stuff on his desk, probably pretending to be busy. I paused.

'Are you OK?' I asked gently, knowing full well that he wasn't. I went over to him and put my arms around him.

'I want to protect you from all this, son, but you're old enough now to understand. This is a big thing I have ahead of me and I'm going to need your help, so I am.' He turned round in his chair and put his arms around my waist, resting his head against me. I couldn't see his face. He did not say a word. I stroked his hair, and it occurred to me at the time how long it was since I had been able to hold him like this. It reminded me of the times when he was six or seven and used to come home with cuts and bruises from playing, or little worries from his day at school. At eighteen he was a pretty cool customer, and rarely liked to show his emotions.

'Things like this can be hard to talk about,' I said, 'but if you want to discuss it anytime I will try to tell you everything I know, and explain as much as I can about what is wrong with me, and what the doctors are doing about it. At the moment, I must say I don't know very much myself.' I waited a moment. All the kids knew how Ger and I felt about telling the truth: honesty was something we were very firm about, and had impressed upon them that no matter what they have done, whatever has happened, the most important thing is to be open and honest.

I grew up in a family where there were many secrets – my father's drinking problem being one of them – and I wanted something better for my own children.

'You and Sarah, you two can handle this. But we must protect little Julie. She doesn't know a thing and I can't have her distraught and confused. She needs to be a normal little girl living a normal life. So I'm going to need your help with her.'

'I know, Mum. I'll try.' His voice was muffled and he was holding on to me for dear life.

'Listen, Rich, I'm only little but I'm a fighter, you know I am. I'm not going to let this thing take me down.'

He looked up at me then, his face contorted with grief. He was trying so hard not to break down in front of me. My heart ached for him – this boy who was not quite a man – his world was falling apart, and he thought his mother was going to die. I felt so guilty, so responsible, thinking Dear God, what have I done to give myself this cancer and take me away from my children who need me so much? Was it getting pregnant with Julie, albeit all those years ago? Was it that desperate prayer to God when Sarah was ill? Tears were pouring down my face – I was so full of sadness not for myself, but for this lad. And the realization struck me at the same time that he loved me with all his being – I was that special to him. It was overwhelming. I don't think I have ever felt closer to him, and I will remember that moment, when I knew my boundless love for him was reflected back, until my dying day. Now, when I meet people who tell me that their only

wish is to do something to help their sick parent, I think of
Richard, and how he must have been feeling that night.

'When this gets tough, Richard, you can cry on my shoulder and
I'll cry on yours.' He nodded, forcing a lop-sided grin, and I
slipped out to get Julie ready for bed.

I hardly slept a wink that night, lying awake and worrying,
unable to get that horrible vision the doctor had conjured up out
of my mind. Feeling my breast, I wondered what it would be like
to feel nothing there, or to feel a new, pretend breast made out
of my back muscle – but without a nipple. I would be like a Play-
Doh person with bits stuck on and pulled off by a clumsy toddler.
For the life of me I could not understand how they could pull a
muscle around from my back, and this weird and puzzling image
frightened me far more than the thought of losing my breast. All
this and worse I turned over and over in my mind in absolute
terror, with horrible imaginings crowding into my restless
dreams. I must have dozed a little, because when I woke up I
found tears spilling out of my half-closed eyes.

The clock said 8 am. It was Saturday morning. Not even twenty-
four hours since the diagnosis and I was alone in the house with
Julie, who was still asleep. Gerard, who was anxious to hold on
to normality, had left for work, as had Sarah and Richard. Maria
was out with some of her students getting some last-minute
things before their flight home. My heart sank as I remembered
what was ahead of me this weekend. My sisters were coming
over early that afternoon, and my mother-in-law was joining us
all that evening. They were all to stay over for Sunday dinner.

I knew there was no way I could put a brave face on things in front of them, and, besides, I would have to start telling people. I could practise on them, maybe.

As I brushed my teeth that morning I looked at myself in the bathroom mirror and tried it out. 'I have something to tell you. I have cancer again. Breast cancer.' The words sounded all wrong, my mouth looked strange saying them. Breast cancer. I stared at my breast – it seemed so ordinary really, just the same as it had always looked – and I tried to imagine the lump under the skin with its cells multiplying, spreading, invading my body. No, that was enough. I screwed my eyes tight shut, blotting out the vision.

Julie appeared in my doorway. My God, Julie. How was I going to hold myself together for her?

'Good morning, Mama. What's for breakfast?' My mind went blank and suddenly I felt dizzy. Breakfast?

I sat down heavily on the bed and realized my palms were sweating and my heart was beating wildly in my chest. Surely I wasn't having a heart attack? My breath was coming in short, shallow bursts.

'Would you go downstairs and switch the television on for the minute, there's a good girl … I'll be down shortly.'

'Yeah, great!' At least she was happy – we never usually let her watch TV in the mornings.

After a few minutes my head cleared. I felt shaky and realized this was no heart attack; it was panic – pure and simple. There was no way I could cope with Julie that morning. Not only was I completely exhausted from the night I'd had, I couldn't trust myself not to break down in front of her.

Slowly I made my way downstairs and started fixing breakfast. I felt my eyelids drooping. I wasn't going to be able to stay awake! My heart started beating heavily again. There was only one person I could think of who would not hesitate to help: Grace.

Her husband Sean answered the phone.

'No, sorry Bernie, she's in the shower at the minute. I'll get her to call you later this morning.' That was a blow.

'OK, that's fine. I hope I didn't wake you. Sorry to bother you.'

'It's no bother. Are you all right, Bernie?'

'Yes! Yes, I'm grand. Thanks anyway Sean, I'll talk to you later. See you.'

Three minutes later the phone rang. It was Grace.

'Sean said something was wrong.' Thank goodness for friends – Sean had obviously guessed there was a reason for the early call. What a relief it was to hear her voice, and everything spilled out of me in a rush. The cancer was back, I was on my own, I couldn't take care of Julie, I was afraid of what was going to happen to us all, I was feeling panicky and out of control.

'I'm coming right over – I'll be with you soon.' Within fifteen minutes she was with me, hair still wet. And, bless her, she stayed all day until the others got back. We chatted about what had happened over the past few days, and she played with Julie while I dozed on the couch; she made me cups of tea, cried with me, brought me chocolate biscuits, and tried to make me laugh. Somehow she knew just what to say, and what not to say. I was so grateful to her for getting me through that first terrible day, when I was still raw with shock.

As it happened, Ger had spared me the necessity of telling Aquinas and Deirdre by phoning them before they came. When they arrived I opened the door to let them in and they both held out their arms to me. My big sisters who had always looked out for me as a kid, plaited my hair, helped dress me, clattered me if I was cheeky – here they were, both devastated by the news, still caring for me in their grown-up sister way.

'You know, then,' I said. They nodded.

'Well, come on in. Julie can't wait to see you.' It was too soon to talk about it.

It was a clear, sunny afternoon and I had prepared drinks for everyone out on the patio. I, still exhausted, went through the motions of entertaining them all, wandering in and out with trays of drinks and plates of food. The best thing for me was see-ing how Julie, normally such a shy child, opened up like a little flower that weekend. I don't know what got into her: perhaps she sensed that I was unable to perform myself, but she rose to the occasion magnificently, entertaining everyone with little dances she had learnt, games and songs and funny stories. I have not seen her behave so confidently either before or since, but she was a true godsend to us all that day.

Apart from her antics there was a lowering atmosphere hanging over the day that reminded me of a funeral. My sisters and Maria would be out on the patio gabbing away – then I would appear with some snacks and their chitter-chatter would instantly stop. Silence. Of course I knew they had been talking about me, and I knew they were worried and all, but it hurt me that they were treating me as if I wasn't there. I felt like I was no longer a per-son, a friend, a sister – but the embodiment of this terrible curse, cancer. It was bigger than me, it cancelled out me. It gave them leave to talk about me, but not with me. This happened several times, and it was the strangest feeling. At some level, though, I suppose I understood that they were just concerned about me, and I knew they thought they were being terribly subtle about it, so I said nothing. But I couldn't wait until the next day when they'd be gone. I had been glad of company but at times that day I just wanted to be on my own.

Later on that afternoon I was sitting on the couch reading to Julie. I had my arms round her and she was snuggled up to me: I was shattered, and she was glad to have her mummy to herself for once that weekend. Before I knew it we were both asleep.

'Wake up, Julie,' I heard Aquinas whispering a little later on. 'Time to go to the party.' I opened my eyes, remembering that Julie did indeed have a birthday party to go to. That was good – it would get her out of the house to do normal kiddy things. I forced myself to get up, and Grace and I took her down the road to her friend's house. When I picked her up a couple of hours later it gladdened my heart to see her racing around the garden with a dozen other excited five-year-olds, splashing through a paddling pool and trying to catch hold of bubbles that an older brother was blowing. This was what she should be doing, and this is what I needed to hang on to for her – sunny days of uncomplicated happiness, free from the shadows that were crowding in on the rest of us.

When Gerard came back after work, bringing his mother with him, we were all ready for something to take us out of ourselves. It was a balmy evening and we all drifted outside with our food and drinks, enjoying the warm weather. We opened bottle after bottle of wine, hardly noticing how much we were drinking. Sarah and Richard were talking together, united and friendly for once. Deirdre's son Terence was there too, enjoying the craic with the two of them. We were all trying to have such fun, and indeed at times I felt almost elated, yet this was anything but a normal family gathering. I sensed a kind of urgency amongst us, a desperate need to feel happy and excited, a need to deny and forget the awful truth that was only just dawning on us. It wasn't like me to drink – a glass of wine with a meal was all I ever had – but once I had started in earnest that night, I couldn't stop. At one point, sick with wine and emotion, I stumbled into the toilet. Overwhelmed with sudden misery, I started sobbing.

Deirdre must have heard me, because I remember her suddenly being there and putting her arms around me.

'I must have done something terrible in my life to deserve this,' I said through my tears. 'It is so unfair. The first time it was easy to be brave, but now I'm just so dreadfully weary of it all. I don't know how I'm going to get through this.'

'You will because you must. You're a survivor – you're so much better than I am at dealing with setbacks.'

'I might die, Deirdre.' She was silent, and I saw tears welling up in her own eyes.

'Don't even say that. It's not going to happen.' I was her baby sister, and it was unthinkable that I might disrupt the natural order of things by getting a fatal illness before my older siblings.

'I just feel so tired, so worn out. I don't know if I have the energy to fight this.'

Deirdre had been to hell and back in her own life and I knew she understood that feeing of impotent fury at the cards life had dealt me. Her husband had died very suddenly at the age of forty-two, completely without warning. It had devastated her and her son, and it took them years to recover from the loss. Sometimes, even now, I suspect she has not yet recovered.

'Listen, I know you, you'll know how to cope. I'm worried about the rest of us, watching you, feeling helpless. You're tough,

Bernadette. I know you can do it.' She buoyed me up as well as she could, until I felt able to go back outside.

I found Aquinas talking with Anne. 'No one else seems to have so much tragedy in their lives. Look what has happened to us: our Dad, my baby, Deirdre's husband, Frank's two wives. What's going on? Why us? What else are we going to be hit by?' Then Gerard broke in:

'I know it looks like that, but I think if you dig a little you will always find something fairly awful in everyone's lives. It's the way people deal with it that counts, I think.' He drew me away a little, not wanting me to be affected by the idea that we had been singled out for destruction by an angry and indiscriminate God.

'We were doing so well, we were all so happy.' I was almost shouting the words. 'This is twisting my mind up, this second cancer. I'm so angry I want to break something.' I kicked a wooden chair and hurt my toe. I was as bitter as hell.

'I know, Bernie. I feel it too. I don't know what to say to make it better for you. All I can say is that I really feel we can get through this, you know. We're both strong, and whenever you're feeling weak I'll be even stronger for you. You know I'll always take care of you, whatever happens.'

He was such a rock to me, I could fit my complaints about him onto the head of a pin. Of course we've had our ups and downs just like any couple, we're not perfect, but I do feel so incredibly fortunate to have Gerard in my life. I don't know if he will ever know how much he did for me over the coming, terrible months. Sarah came over. 'Mum, I hope you don't mind, I told my friends.' Christ, she had loads of friends. Did the entire village know by now?

'Oh. Who?'

'Um, Ciara, and Emily, and Jessica. Is that OK?'

I nodded. Of course I minded, but I understood. Her mother had cancer, she needed to talk it through with her friends. It was no secret, and that was important. This must not become a taboo subject.

The evening wore on, and we all got completely plastered, each one of us using alcohol as a way of blotting out reality. I can't remember going to bed; in fact I think Ger carried me upstairs that night.

The last thing I remember is sinking under the covers and craving the sweet oblivion of sleep. If only I did not have to face a tomorrow.

Chapter Fourteen

'Battle-Stations, Mum!'

⤵

I woke up the next morning with a throbbing head. It hurt to open my eyes and my mouth felt like a small furry animal had made a nest in it. I groaned: I had not been hung over like this for many years, and now I remembered why.

'Water ... orange juice,' I croaked at Ger, who wasn't in much better shape himself. What a night we'd had – much of it was a blur now, but I knew I'd never felt so happy, or so wretched, at any one time. *It was the best of times, it was the worst of times.* Charles Dickens' well-worn phrase now had a new meaning for me. I swallowed a glass of water and shut my eyes again. Go away, day.

Richard popped his head around the door. 'Mum? Dad? You two all right? I'm just getting Julie her breakfast.' I sat up and smiled at him, much as it brought a searing pain to my temples. Richard was such a great son, I thought. We were so lucky he seemed to have bypassed the much-dreaded stroppy teenager phase and cruised straight through to responsible young man. And at his age he had the capacity to shrug off a night's drinking more easily than us.

'Will I get you a bit of breakfast?'

'Er … no thanks,' mumbled Gerard. 'We'll be up soon and we'll be going to Mass in an hour so could you make sure everyone's up and ready? Thanks, Rich.' Richard nodded and disappeared. Ger sank back into the pillows and massaged his temples. 'I feel like I've been poisoned.'

'You have! Think how toxic alcohol must be if it makes you feel this bad. I think our bodies are trying to tell us something.' How I hated feeling like this. I had to get ready to face the day. The second day, as I thought of it. It was now forty-eight hours since my diagnosis and it was starting to sink in properly.

Later that morning, at Mass, I knelt with my family in our usual place. I was trying to concentrate on the reading, but the priest's sing-song voice washed over me, the smell of incense was soporific and my mind wandered. I remembered going to Mass as a child, every Sunday without fail – my mother was very devout. It was a special outing for us kids: having worn our school uniform all week we would wear our best clothes to church and try to behave as quietly and sensibly as possible. Half the town would be there – it was the kind of place where everyone knew, or thought they knew, everybody else's business. We were friendly to our neighbours and played in the street with the local kids, but nobody really knew our business. We didn't wash our dirty linen in public, my fiercely proud Mum would say, not us. They would not have known how alone she felt with a houseful of growing kids and a husband who drank too much; they would not have known the reasons that drove my dad to drink most of his wages, or indeed why his own father had behaved in the same way. Only she and God knew the truth.

Dad went to a different church in the middle of the town, near to where he grew up. Sometimes, if I was lucky, he would take me with him. 'This is my youngest,' he would say, showing me off to his friends. And I would swell with pride as I sat next to him, admiring his smoothed-down hair and clean jacket – even if the big hands that held mine were rough and grey from the building work he might have been fortunate enough to have been given that week. I used to ask Dad if God was watching me all the time, or only when I was in church. 'All the time, lassie, all the time.'

As we all stood up to sing the offertory hymn, Julie standing up on the pew itself, I glanced sideways at my sister Deirdre. Did she believe now as fervently as we all did as children? Back then we lived in terror of hell-fire and damnation, but of course we never did anything that could be classified as a mortal sin. I used to trail off to confession with her on Saturdays, prepared to confess my regular sin: 'I stole the sugar.' I knew it was definitely a sin because my mother had told me so. Once I used a bold word and Mum frightened the life out of me by telling me it was a mortal sin. We lived our lives on simple precepts: Do as you would be done by. What goes around comes around. Tell the truth, help others, serve God. I knew that if I was good I would go to Heaven. If not, the Other Place. God could be fierce and vengeful, so I did my best to stay on the straight and narrow.

Well, I thought bitterly, my anger of the night before starting to resurface, I had probably not lived an entirely blameless life but I hadn't done anything to deserve such a bad deal. All I wanted to do was raise my little family. I wasn't a bad person and nor was anyone in my family – were we all being punished for crimes we hadn't committed? Deirdre was singing her heart out next to me. She couldn't have been a better person, and look what God had brought down upon her head. I remembered once telling our priest – who had innocently come to the house on a duty visit – that I wasn't so sure I believed in Heaven and Hell. My mother was ready to kill me, and that priest was out of the house before giving me an answer. 'That's funny,' I had said to her as he disappeared through the door, 'I thought he was supposed to know about this stuff.'

Perhaps, I thought to myself as we all drove back home in silence that day, my fourteen-year-old self had been right to question it all. At that moment it truly felt as if I was existing in a Godless universe. There was no guiding providence, no purpose, no point. All we pitiful humans had was ourselves. Then nothing.

As soon as we got home I took my hangover back to bed for a while, grateful that Anne and Ger were preparing Sunday dinner. I needed some time by myself to think. What was ahead of me? Was there anything I could do? Something, anything, to improve this desperate situation. What did I need to know about it? I had some health books on my shelf which I had studiously avoided ever since that nurse had told me not to read anything. Aw feck it, I thought, I've got to start somewhere. I decided I wasn't going to go through whatever treatment was meted out to me blindly and acceptingly. This was my body, and my mind. I had to find out if there was anything I could do to deal with this. I'll do what I'm told, I thought; I'm not going to challenge the medical system, but perhaps there are other ways. I was clutching at straws, and I knew it. Where to begin, I had no idea. I picked up one book, almost at random. It was *Spontaneous Healing* by Andrew Weil, and it had a whole section on cancer. An hour later I was still reading it, and was already starting to feel more positive. I read about all the different ways I could increase my 'internal resistance' and help my body to heal. I read about cranial osteopathy, visualization, herbs, tonics, healing foods, supplements, yoga, and more. I read miraculous stories of ordinary people somehow switching on their bodies' natural defence systems and recovering fully from fatal diseases. It was as if someone from outside the rigid confines of the medical world might just be granting me a reprieve: maybe I wasn't bound to die from this thing after all. This book, and many others that I read over the next months, gave me huge hope and encouragement: people do get better. When your back's against the wall, it's amazing how you can find a way.

A shout roused me: dinner-time. On my way downstairs I looked in on Richard.

'Richard!' I said excitedly, waving the book at him. 'Listen. I'm discovering that there are loads of things I can do to help myself. It's all here in this book – I just need to find out what it is going to take for me to boost my body's own defences.'

He grinned at me. 'Battle-stations, Mum!' he said, punching me on the shoulder. He had caught my mood exactly. I was ready to fight rather than take it lying down.

'That's right,' I rejoined, 'No surrender!' We went down together, suddenly crazily full of hope.

If the rest of the family were surprised to see us laughing and chatting as we sat down for the meal no one commented on it, but the atmosphere suddenly lifted, as if everyone heaved a collective sigh of relief. I could still not think of anything else, though, and at one point I found myself saying, 'I'm probably going to lose all my hair.'

'You'll have to get a wig,' said Anne, Ger's mother. 'They have lovely ones nowadays.'

'Oh no, I think if it started to fall out I wouldn't hide it with a wig or a scarf – I'd go the whole hog and shave the lot off,' I said. Sarah spluttered into her gravy.

'Well, it worked for Demi Moore, Mum – she could be your role model.'

'Yeah, I'd look great in a white T-shirt and a pair of combats.' Everyone laughed, and I felt as if things were really not so bad after all. We had a happy day after that, and at the end of the day my sisters and mother-in-law left in good spirits.

But I felt drained after that weekend, and wanted nothing more than an early night. I was just thinking about going up for a bath when Sarah got back from Jessica's house. She had been with her friends and had that look on her face which meant she wanted to talk.

'Mum, I hope you don't mind, I told the lads tonight.' Oh Jesus, I thought, the boys know now. Breast cancer was a woman's thing, I felt. Now if they met me in the street they would be looking at me, and imagining me without a breast. It was a silly thing, but somehow it mattered. Sarah must have realized I was unhappy about this and tears sprang to her eyes.

'I'm sorry, I just needed to tell my friends. I don't know how to deal with this – I'm so frightened for you ... Mum, what's going to happen to you?' she sat down on the couch and covered her eyes.

'Sarah, Sarah, love. It doesn't have to be bad. Come here to me.' I wrapped her in my arms and spent the next two hours doing my best to talk her around. I told her what I had told Richard two nights before: that I needed her help, that we needed to protect our little Julie, and that I would tell her all I could. All the while she was sobbing her heart out, her head on my shoulder. I knew she had to do this – this was her way, and I felt it was right for me to let her grieve that night with me. I have seen what holding in fear and sorrow does to a person and I wanted her to feel free to let it all out then, at the beginning. I helped her into bed that night, my beautiful girl, both of us spent with crying. I kissed her swollen eyelids.

'I promise you, Sarah, if you want to come and talk to me about any of this, at any time, I'll be here to listen. I'm your mum and I love you beyond belief. None of that is going to change just because I'm sick.'

My God, look how I was hurting these two children, and the treatment had not even started yet. I hated to see them so worried and frightened, and to know that I was the cause of their pain. At least Julie had been spared this ordeal.

Two days later I had an appointment with the surgeon – the one who had done the needle biopsy – who was to perform the operation. He was just back from holiday but my oncologist was still away. 'These guys!' Ger complained, 'They're always jetting off on holiday.' He came with me that day, but this time I was the one in charge. From all the reading I had done over the past couple of days I was determined not to go in blind, and had come armed with a list of questions.

'What are we dealing with here?' I began. 'I need to know how big this tumour is, and what stage it is at.' As I carried on, questioning the surgeon about secondaries, and about my lymph glands, Ger raised his eyebrows quizzically at me, as if to say 'How do you know all this?' For his part, the surgeon had all the answers at his fingertips, but was flummoxed only by one thing I said:

'The other surgeon I saw on Friday when you were away said I would need a total mastectomy and a new breast made of back muscle tissue.' I said this without flinching but I saw him do a double take.

'Oh no, no. That's reconstruction, that's much further down the line. We don't need to be thinking about things like that at this point. Let's deal with the job in hand. Put all that out of your mind.' He was clearly appalled to hear what I had been told, but he managed to maintain his professional dignity as well as making me feel calmer about my prospects.

'You have two options,' he said, getting out a piece of paper on which he started to draw a diagram. 'Number one: we remove the breast, you have radiation therapy but no chemotherapy. Number two: we remove the lump with a 2cm margin around it, you have twenty-five radiation sessions and six months of chemo. The drawback is that if there are any cancer cells in the margin around the tumour we would have to go back in and remove the entire breast.'

We discussed these options at length, and I realized that I was to be allowed to choose.

'My instinct,' I said to them both, 'is to have the whole breast removed and be done with it. What do you think, Ger?'

'I don't know, Bernie, it's your body. I think you need to spend a few days thinking about this.'

'That's right. Whatever you decide, we'll operate on Friday. Go and see your oncologist on Thursday to discuss it and see what he thinks.' There was not much time – this was already Tuesday. We left the surgeon's office, me clutching the little drawing he did for me. I still have it in my desk, a little reminder of that fearful and uncertain time.

When I got home I called my friend Siobhan, who I knew had had a mastectomy eight years earlier. I outlined my two options to her. 'Why don't you come over for a cuppa and we can have a good chat about it then,' she said.

She is an incredibly positive woman, and had obviously recovered well from her bout with cancer. We chatted about her operation, and how she came to make the decision, but when she opened her blouse for me I had to stifle a gasp of horror. A thick white scar slashed diagonally across the space where her breast had been. It looked unnatural, painful, wrong. The skin was puckered, and even eight years on it looked ugly and deformed. I lowered my eyes. Mother of God.

'Perfectly OK, isn't it?' Siobhan commented. 'I'm totally happy walking around the house naked. My husband calls me his Amazonian woman after those female hunters who cut their right boobs off so they can use their bows and arrows properly.'

'What about going swimming?' I ventured to ask.

'Oh, well I usually go already changed. I've got a prosthesis, a falsie, and a special swimsuit. And of course there are changing rooms so I don't offend anyone when I get changed afterwards. It's not a problem.'

The fear of cancer killing me was greater than the fear of losing a breast, but as a woman I just couldn't bear the idea of looking like this, of feeling like a freak, of always feeling I should cover up rather than risk horrifying or embarrassing anyone. I was grateful for Siobhan's honesty and willingness to show me her scar. I just hoped that my oncologist would recommend the other option.

'Statistics show absolutely no difference in recovery rates,' was what he did say. He was back in his office, incongruously glowing with health after his long break. I knew him well, but was in no mood for idle chit-chat about his holiday. I felt weak, pale and exhausted after days of going over the two options in my mind.

'I'm worried that if I have the lumpectomy there will still be cancer cells in the margin and then I'm back where I started, except I'll have had an extra pointless operation.'

'It can be very distressing for women to lose their breast, in my experience,' he said thoughtfully. 'We know that it is primary cancer – as yet there are no secondaries, although we will have to take away some lymph glands. I have to say that, given the identical recovery rates, I'd recommend a lumpectomy. But this is your decision.'

'What would you recommend if it was your wife?'

'Lumpectomy.'

I was enormously relieved and reassured to hear this, and to think I did not necessarily have to lose the breast. So I opted for the lumpectomy, and the operation was set for the very next day. I would have three weeks to recover, provided the 'margin' was clear, then the chemo would start, with the twenty-five radiation sessions when the chemo was well under way.

This was it then, I thought, as we drove home from the hospital that day. I was going to have to be strong. It was a cliché, but I knew now why people talked about their 'fight' with cancer. It was my enemy and I was going to have to confront it with all the weapons in my armoury.

If you have read this far you will know by now the kind of woman I am – no health freak, no scientific genius, not even particularly well educated. Just an ordinary Irish woman faced with the terrifying possibility of dying before my children grew up. Someone who loved life and wanted to hang on to it. The one thing I could do was read, and read I did from that point onwards as if my life depended on it. I read selectively at first, avoiding books on chemotherapy and radiation because I was not yet ready to know about the gory details. I took it one step at a time, absorbing what I could. I started to find out about lectures and talks, and I began to make notes; the notes became a file and the file became a library. The mass of information I was accumulating was in some ways mind-boggling and in other ways mind-expanding, but my need to understand what was happening to me – and what I could do about it – was overwhelming.

Every few weeks from that point on, Richard would repeat to me our special battle-cry, 'Battle-stations, Mum!' and although I would ask him not to whack me on my arm again, it made me feel so tough.

It was a toughness and inner resilience I would need over the coming months more than I could ever have imagined.

Chapter Fifteen

Cruel and Unusual

⁓

'If you're really lucky I'll give you my underpants too,' quipped Ger.

He and I were in the hospital waiting for the nurse to come in and start to prepare me for the lumpectomy operation. My friend Grace had come with us and had kindly offered to collect a load of Ger's shirts to take home to iron. She was pretending to complain about them – some of them were pure cotton and took ages to press properly. The silly, nervous banter between them took my mind off what I was about to undergo. Then the nurse appeared with a gown for me to put on, and briskly set about making me ready. I started to shiver even though it was not cold.

I was not only nervous, I was bone tired too: I had been up late the night before making a dress for Julie. She was to be the flower girl at my nephew Darren's wedding, and I knew that if I didn't get it finished before my operation I might not have the strength in my arms afterwards. 'Leave it, Bernie,' begged his fiancée Lisa. 'You've enough on your plate. I'll buy a dress – we've still got a couple of weeks. Please don't worry.' But I was determined: I had the material – clouds of beautiful cream

chiffon and wine silk for a sash. Sitting in our kitchen that afternoon looking at Julie, and knowing what was ahead of me, I
realized that making the dress would stop me from breaking
down in front of her. So while Richard played with her, I knocked
sparks out of my machine and sat up late sewing dozens of tiny
wine-coloured silk flowers onto the prettiest little dress you could
imagine.

As I lay on the trolley the next day, waiting for the nurses to take
me down to the operating theatre, it was a vision of little Julie
trying on her dress that morning that I held in my mind. 'Oh,
Mama,' she had breathed, scarcely able to contain her delight. 'I
will look like a real fairy.'

'That's my girl,' said Ger to me as I was wheeled into the operating theatre. He was trying to smile encouragingly, but what I read
on his face was fear.

Hours later, I was aware that I was coming to. I heard the soft
noises of the ward, and the bleeping of the machines. A television
was on somewhere. I was sore under my left arm but I didn't
want to dwell on that right now. I lay there for a bit, just thinking. Gradually I opened my eyes, and the first thing I saw was
Ger gazing down at me with such a tender expression. What was
this doing to my poor man? I wondered, feeling terrible for giving him all this worry.

'Hello there,' I murmured. He smiled and reached for my right
hand, giving it a little squeeze. We were silent for a time, until I
stupidly asked him what he was thinking. Poor love, he wasn't

going to tell me the truth – that here he was, looking at his little wife who could be heading for an early grave.

'Your breath stinks,' he said. Good old Ger, I thought, deflecting gloomy thoughts as always.

'Have you seen the surgeon?' All I could think about was the all-important margin around the lump, and whether it would be found to contain any cancer cells.

'Yes, he's doing his rounds. I expect he'll be along later.' And he was.

'Tell me,' I said urgently to him when he reached my bed, although I was still woozy from the anaesthetic: 'Was the margin clear?' He smiled sympathetically.

'There's time enough for that. We won't have the results for a few days. You concentrate on getting better. The operation went as well as could be expected.'

Huh, I thought to myself. I won't be able to recover from this operation if I have to be rushed back in for a mastectomy. So each time the surgeon appeared on his rounds I asked him the same question. I was obsessed with this damn margin.

Over the next few days I was inundated with visitors. I was glad to see them, but I was in too much pain to talk much. It's a funny thing, being in hospital. People want to see you, or at least they want to show you that they care enough to come and see you, and in a way you want to see them too, except you don't want them to see you looking awful and you're not really up to small talk. It is such an artificial environment that after a few minutes they run out of things to say and you wait for them to go so that you can go back to the strange half-life of the ward: a parallel universe in which you lie helplessly while needles are put into your arms or legs, and drips are taken out and monitors monitored, and all you have to do is watch the clock and wait for the results of whatever test or operation you have had.

I did want to see the kids, though, and my heart leapt when I first saw them walk into the ward. Julie ran up to me and flung her arms over the bed covers. Too late I realized that just next to where she was standing was the bottle collecting the blood draining from the incision. Before I could say anything she cried out in disgust, 'Mama, you're bleeding!'

'I know, pet, don't worry though – it doesn't hurt. It's just where I had the operation – that blood needs to come out to stop it getting infected. It's helping me get better.'

'Oh, OK.' She accepted my explanation without a murmur, and busied herself with laying out some cards and pictures she had been making me. I hoped this image of dripping blood wouldn't stay with her.

'Can't you sit up, Mama?' she asked. I tried, but my arm was still hurting too much. The skin around my breast, and under my arm where the lymph glands had been, was clamped with staples rather than stitches, to seal the skin after the surgeon's knife had gone in, and the tightness meant I could hardly move my arm. The physiotherapist had been in several times to try to get me to do some exercises: I had found them almost impossible but I knew I had to keep trying. It took weeks to regain full mobility in that arm, and in fact my underarm is still sore from the scar tissue. For a long time it felt like I had pins and needles, and I would shake the arm as if to get the blood moving again, to get the feeling back. It never came back entirely – I am still numb on the back of my arm where the nerves were cut. It is something I have just had to get used to.

It was my oncologist, in the end, who managed to get me the results of the tests on the margin around the excised lump. It was clear of cancer cells, thanks be to God. I felt I had come very close to the wire this time, but the knowledge I had made the right decision on the operation made me feel good.

I arrived back home to find the house full of flowers. Everywhere I looked there were vases, jugs, bowls, crammed with roses, lilies, gerberas, peonies and many flowers I did not know the names of. They were absolutely beautiful and smelt heavenly, and I felt strengthened by all these good wishes – but it reminded me of a funeral parlour (or perhaps I am just not used to getting flowers!). The doorbell went constantly, and the phone was rarely quiet, with people offering support and asking if there was anything they could do. Neighbours, friends, parents of my children's friends – these were the people, I knew, who would be at my funeral. I know it sounds morbid, but these are the kinds of thoughts that come into your head when you are told you have cancer. It was not just me – countless people have told me of this feeling that they can picture their funeral. During days like these, when I was too sick to be involved in day-to-day life, I was acutely aware of the love with which I was surrounded, and I know how fortunate I am to have felt this.

A few days later my entire arm inflated like a rugby ball. This was a fairly common condition called lymphodoema – a swelling that often happens to post-operative patients – but I had neither been warned about it, nor was I prepared for the pain. When my friend Patricia called in to see me that day I remember saying, 'Christ, will you stick a pin in this arm? I have got to relieve this appalling pressure.' She didn't do that, but she did call the hospital for me.

'The sister on duty said to come back in if it doesn't improve. Apparently lots of people get this and it does get better eventually.' Not much help from them, then.

Patricia was so kind to me that day, for when she realized I was in utter agony she spent the rest of the day gently massaging the arm. I found eventually that if I raised it up I did get some relief, perhaps because the fluid drained back. The next day it was back to normal, and all the pain of the previous day had evaporated into thin air.

This was just as well, because Grace had promised to call to help me pick out something to wear for Darren and Lisa's wedding the following weekend. We tried to find something that was light enough for the warm summer weather, but that also covered enough of my arms so as not to show my stitches. I could barely lift my arm with the staples holding the incision together, but we managed to find something in the end. My nephew Darren is very special to me, and his wedding was the best I have ever been to.

I felt like the belle of the ball. Everyone said they wanted to dance with me – nephews, cousins, in-laws, the lot – and Sarah never left my side all night. We had such fun; I had never been in so much demand! Ger and I were dancing at one point when Richard came up and gently took over. What a gorgeous feeling it is to dance with your son – this boy you have held as a baby and watched grow into a strapping lad, and now a fine young man. I was so made up over this, so proud. If my life had ended then and there I would have died the happiest woman in Ireland.

I was getting a glass of water, hot from all the dancing, when Deirdre came up. 'Look at you!' she exclaimed. 'No one can believe how well you are doing.' Of course, this is why I was suddenly Miss Popularity: I was the person with the death sentence, and this was their last chance to have a turn on the dance-floor with Bernadette.

'Oh, for goodness sake, I'm not dead yet, you know,' I laughed. I made light of it, but it was indeed a strange place to be in. Pushed into the limelight despite myself, set apart from the others by my illness, regarded as someone slightly special, slightly marked, a ticking time-bomb waiting to go off. The person about whom others said, 'There but for the grace of God …' and felt lucky to be themselves. Oh feck it, I thought, putting all this out of my head. I might as well get on and enjoy myself. Occasions like this were going to be few and far between, for my chemotherapy sessions were due to start soon.

The lymphodoema had been painful, but nothing in my life so far had prepared me for the unimaginable cruelty of chemotherapy.

'Mama's got to go into hospital again today, pet,' I explained to Julie one morning.

'Will you be back after school?' she asked.

'No, Mama will be staying in hospital for two days, but don't worry, you'll have Dada and Richard and Sarah to take care of you.'

As I stood at the nurses' station at the front of the now familiar ward later that day, waiting for them to allocate me a bed, I saw a woman who was pushing a drip on a stand. She was shuffling along to the lavatories, making very slow progress. I smiled as she trundled past me, and she stopped. She had thin mousey hair and almost transparent skin, and she could barely lift her head up.

'I'm Eileen,' she said. I think she could see I was terrified, and in her own way thought she could make me feel better, even though she herself was so sick. 'My family is coming in to see me – you might see them, three fine boys! Tell them I'll be back in a few minutes.' I told her I had three children too. Before she went into the toilet she said softly, 'You're going to be fine. Good luck, love.'

Just then my oncologist entered the ward, and I heard him speak to her. 'Please,' I heard her plead, 'don't give me any more chemo, I can't take any more. The last lot almost killed me.' She can't take any more chemo, I thought. Look at the state of her, poor woman. And here I was, about to embark on my first session. It did not exactly inspire me: it filled me with dread.

To prepare me for the first chemotherapy injection I had a shot of steroids. These were really trippy, making me hallucinate – I saw people becoming taller and wider as if I was looking in those weird mirrors you see at theme parks. I shrank away from the walls as I imagined objects falling down on me – I was frightened and alienated. Then a nurse approached wielding an enormous needle – at least it seemed enormous to me – attached to a huge vial of clear liquid. She had surgical gloves on, and I found out later why. This chemical is so toxic that if it is spilt on naked skin it will burn a hole right in the flesh. If it accidentally drips onto the floor it is treated almost like a leak of nuclear waste. This was what was going directly into my bloodstream, in three separate injections, taking half an hour in all. This was what was going to kill the cancer cells – and a lot else besides. This first session I treated in a fairly matter-of-fact way, but the time I came in for the next ones I started shaking the moment the needle went in, for I knew what was ahead of me.

'This stuff plays havoc with your immune system. Stay away from supermarkets and crowds around the seventh to the tenth days – you don't want to come down with any nasty bugs.' Oh God, I thought. Julie's always coming home from school with coughs and sneezes. 'And another thing, Bernadette,' she continued, as she smoothed a plaster onto the bleeding point where the needle entered. 'One of the side effects of chemotherapy is that it can push you into an early menopause.' She left me then – I was staying in for two nights while they monitored my reaction to the chemo – and it took a while for what she had just said to sink in. As if having breast cancer wasn't enough – here I was now about to lose my fertility too. Not that I wanted any more children, but Aquinas had had a terrible time with 'the change', and this seemed to add insult to injury.

I lay there waiting to be sick, as I had heard I would be. Nothing. Eventually I nodded off, and when I woke I saw Gerard coming towards me. Except it didn't look like him – it was a ten-foot high version of him. I was frightened and tried to sit up, but the bed seemed to be moving. I held onto the sides and cried out, feeling him put his hand on my shoulder to calm me. The steroids again – I hated feeling like this. I still showed no signs of sickness, and two days later I was told I could go home.

Before I left I was given a bone scan to ascertain whether the cancerous cells had reached my bone marrow. This I thought was fairly routine and I went through the procedure, drinking that horrible drink in something of a daze – until the radiographer dropped her bombshell.

'Because of this scan you will be essentially radioactive for a day or so. Don't go too near any children or anyone pregnant for twenty-four hours.' I couldn't believe it. This was all I needed – how do you explain that to a five-year-old who has not seen her mother for two days?

As I left the nurse handed me some tablets. 'These are for any sickness you might experience,' she explained. I looked at them and recognized the packet. I had taken them before for motion sickness (I have always been a bad traveller) and felt encouraged – perhaps I would not be feeling too bad after all. I could surprise Julie and be there for her tea. How wrong I was.

I stumbled through my front door and had to cling to the hall table – it seemed as if the coats were falling off their hooks on to me. Scared, and wanting these strange feelings to stop, I went to bed and tried to sleep. But that evening I started to vomit, and could not stop. I vomited and vomited, bent double over the loo. I vomited until I thought I could vomit no more, and still it went on. Each time I felt my stomach rising I could hear myself swearing. Was that me? I was coming out with foul words I hardly thought I knew. Sarah must have heard me, for she came into the bathroom at one point. 'Mum! You look awful. What can I do?' She came over and held my hair back while I retched. She was so gentle, her love for me shining through when I desperately needed her most. Then Julie came up. 'Are you sick, Mama?' I could see she was frightened.

'Yes, a little,' I managed to stammer. 'Don't you worry, I'll be better later. Go play in your room for a while and Sarah will be with you shortly.' I edged away from her, anxious not to zap her with my radioactive body. But she lingered, reluctant to leave me, and curious too. Being sick was something of an event in our family, and Julie was always eager to be involved. I knew she wanted a hug – she hated seeing me ill. Eventually I persuaded Sarah to take her away and occupy her. 'I'll be fine up here by myself for a while. Hand me a cold flannel before you go. Oh, and give Dad a call, will you?'

When Ger came home he could not believe the state of me. He knelt beside me in the bathroom and stroked my hair. 'God, Bernie, what have they done to you? How are you going to make it through another seven sessions of this?'

'I'll do it because I have to. What else can I do?' I said through gritted teeth. He was called away to the phone, and for what seemed like hours I stayed bowed over the toilet bowl, still suffering from the strange effects of the steroids, not really knowing where I was or how long I had been there, unable to do anything other than vomit and wait for it to stop. My every instinct told me this could not be good for me.

That night Ger and Sarah put Julie to bed. She asked them to send me in to kiss her goodnight, but fortunately she was so tired that she didn't make a fuss when they told her I was busy. I continued throwing up non-stop all through the night and into the following morning.

It turned out that the telephone call Ger had taken that evening was from a woman I had met in the hospital a few weeks before. Her daughter had been through chemotherapy, and I had told her when I was due to start the treatment. With the unerring instinct for empathy that only those who have been through this particular mill display, she called because she knew there would be someone in our house who would need to talk to someone who knew.

'I have never opened up to a stranger like that before,' admitted Ger to me the next day. 'I told her everything – she really seemed to understand.' That was when I realized that Ger needed as much support as I did, although it was of a different kind. Like many men he did not find it easy to ask for help, but when it was offered he accepted it gratefully.

The following day I was still being sick. I had a raging thirst, but all I could keep down were sips of green tea. It was a Saturday, and I was so thankful to be able to rely on Sarah's help with Julie, who appeared in my room that morning looking anxious.

'Are you better yet, Mama? Can we have a cuddle?' As she came close to the bed I cried out in alarm.

'No, honey! Mama has had a special treatment that means it isn't safe for you to touch me for a while.' They had told me one day, but I thought I should leave it two, just to make certain.

'Can I sit on your lap?'

'Not until tomorrow. We'll have lots of cuddles then.' She turned away unhappily. Damn this bloody chemo, I muttered angrily to myself.

Richard, meanwhile, was away on holiday with his friends in Greece. When he had realized that it would coincide with my starting the chemo he immediately offered to stay home, but I would not hear of it. I felt sure it was important for him to carry on as normal and insisted he went off as planned. I should have guessed that he would call, but when the phone rang as I sat in bed that morning with a sick bowl on my knees I reached over automatically to answer it.

'Mum, it's Rich. Are you OK?' Oh no! How can I hold it together to talk to him now? Sarah suddenly appeared at the door, mouthing *Give me the phone!*

'Well, I'm all right,' I said, trying to talk in a normal voice, willing myself not to vomit.

'What about the chemo? Are you sick with it? How has it made you feel?'

'A little queasy on and off, a little bit sick you know, but I'm grand. Anyway, that's one down, only seven to go.' I wondered if he knew I was lying.

Don't you dare throw up all over the bed! I'm not clearing it up! Sarah was furiously miming her distress. I knew I had to finish the call. I also knew she would clear up anything, no questions asked.

'Are you having a good time?' I asked, determined to have a normal conversation. Richard chatted on about his holiday while I sat, head bowed over the bowl, and eventually I managed to say goodbye.

'You can't carry on like this,' said Sarah the next day, all bossy. 'Phone the hospital and tell them what's happening.' So I did, and I told the nurse on duty that I just couldn't keep up the vomiting.

'Oh!' she said, sounding surprised. 'What are you taking for it?' I named the drug. 'That works for some people, but really I'm afraid vomiting is a very common side effect of chemotherapy. We normally start people off on the lowest dose to see how well they tolerate it. I expect you'll find that after four days or so the sickness will wear off.' Wear off? I thought angrily, it will wear me out.

Exhausted from the vomiting, still at sixes and sevens from the steroids, and desperate to feel clean again, I ran myself a bath. As I got in, Julie's little face appeared around the bathroom door. 'Can I get in with you?' she begged.

'Of course you can, hop in.' We splashed around for fifteen minutes or so when suddenly I remembered. The bone scan. I went cold – the water would be full of radiation. Sweet Jesus, how could I have been so stupid?

'Julie, get out. Come on, quick smart – let's get out.'

'Why, Mama? What's wrong?'

'Just move!' I almost screamed. I plonked her on the bathmat and threw a towel at her. 'Sarah?' I yelled. 'Can you take Julie a minute?' Still wet, I rang the hospital in a panic. They reassured me that it would be fine, but I could not believe them, questioning them again and again. 'Are you sure, are you absolutely positively sure? I'm up to ninety over this!'

Feeling relieved, but not entirely reassured, I got dressed and went to see to Julie. Sarah said she had shut herself in her bedroom and would not let her in. That is where I found her, tidying her room. This was not typical – she was very much a normal five-year-old, and tidying up did not come naturally to her. Yet there she was, Lego miraculously back in its box, books on the shelf and all her soft toys on the bed in a neat row. As I went in she was picking up beads and replacing them in a basket. If I was a psychologist I might have thought that she was perhaps hoping that by imposing order on her own small world she would be able to make the chaos around her disappear. Or that by being 'good' she would be rewarded with a mummy who was well and happy again. For some reason I suddenly remembered an imaginary friend I had invented as a child – I would often be found at the end of the road, my little suitcase packed, running away to stay with 'Catriona'. What a complex life of the mind little children lead.

'What's wrong, love?' I asked. She said nothing, and just shook her head.

'Come on, you can tell me. What is it?'

'I don't know,' came a very small voice.

'You don't like Mama being so sick, is that it?'

At that, she burst into tears, made as if to rush towards me, then stepped back and threw herself on her pillows. I sat on her bed and tried to gather her into my arms.

'Don't, Mama! You said you were not allowed to touch me!' Of course, I suddenly copped on. The poor little mite – as if her world hadn't been shaken enough with me going into hospital, the strange atmosphere in the house, her mother throwing up not just once but constantly, when all she wanted was to be cuddled and comforted and to be told everything was going to be all right. The very thing I had been forbidden to give her was what she needed more than anything else. It had been two days – surely that was enough now.

'Julie, pet, that time is over now. I know it has been hard – I need a cuddle from you too. Listen, sit up on my knee and tell me all about it. There's nothing like a good cry in your Mama's arms.'

She lay on me then, and cried and cried. I held her while her small body was wracked with sobs, her tears soaking into my shirt. 'It's OK, everything will be fine, don't you worry,' I murmured repeatedly, kissing her head, smoothing her tears away with my fingertips. 'Mama's sick at the moment, but I will get better. I need to go to hospital a few more times, and the medicine that makes me better also makes me feel sick.' I tried hard to put it as simply as I could, and gradually her sobs subsided. I wondered then if I should have sent her to stay with her grandmother Anne for those early chemo days. My little pet, still only a baby, having to deal with all this: no matter how hard we tried to protect her, we could not keep all of it away from her. Now when I think about it I think we did the right thing. Yes, she was frightened, and yes – she saw me sicker than I have ever been. She dealt with her fear, and came through to the other side. She saw me at my worst, and she saw me gradually get better. I feel proud that we stayed together as a family through those awful dark days, and I was so heartened to see how Julie gained strength and character over that difficult year.

Still I continued to read and read, determined to find answers. Surely it was more than a coincidence that so many of these books mentioned juicing as the best way to give your body massive amounts of the anti-oxidant vitamins, as well as the vital minerals it needed for recovery? I had to sit up and take notice. I found an old juicing machine I had bought years before when Leslie Kenton had made raw juice fashionable. It didn't work very well, and was difficult to clean, but it was a start. ('Not that again,' groaned Ger). I was starting to suspect that traditional medicine might not hold all of the answers. Next I heard about some digestive enzymes that were widely available in health-food stores – they would enable me to digest more effectively the little amounts of food I was able to keep down. I tried them immediately. Chemotherapy weakens the whole digestive system, and until then anything I ate sat in my stomach like a block of cement; with the enzymes I felt a dramatic difference and I was able to eat without a problem.

I had only just embarked on my course of eight chemotherapy sessions – a treatment that felt utterly barbaric – but simultaneously I was already starting to discover ways of treating myself, because I had to. Slowly but surely, a new dawn seemed to break. It seemed that there might be simple things I could do that would not only ease my way through the chemotherapy, but *also* help me recover from the cancer itself. Bolstered by these new thoughts, I became determined to save my own life, and I felt sure I could see the way forward. This was my chance: probably my one and only chance. It was going to be a rocky road, but one that I did not flinch from following from this point on. As I saw it, I had a choice. To do as I was told and wait and see whether I lived or died. Or to do as I was told and also find out everything I could about how to save my life. And – most of all – carry it through.

Chapter Sixteen

Changing Over

'**O**ne down, seven to go,' my friend Patricia said to me after that first session.

Such a simple phrase, but to me it was as if I was being asked to go mountain climbing without oxygen, ice picks or cold-weather gear. Each one, I felt, was going to be a separate peak to scale, each with different problems, different reactions, and I knew that my immune system would steadily become weaker as each blast of chemo took its toll. The very first session had been shocking in its newness, although in a sense there was something to be said for not knowing what to expect.

'Patricia, it's only August. I won't be through this until next February or March. I just don't want to think about those seven sessions, let alone the twenty-five radiations – whenever they start.' It was best for me not to try to imagine the unimaginable. What I was focussing on was life after chemotherapy. I held this Promised Land in my mind throughout the following months, planning what I was going to do afterwards. 'When all this is behind me', I kept saying. 'When life returns to normal.' The thought that I might be dying I kept to the darkest recesses of my mind, willing myself to focus on my belief that – horrendous as it was – the chemo was killing the cancer cells.

When I went into the hospital for my second chemotherapy session three weeks to the day after the first one, I was afraid, but I was forewarned. I had a brief appointment with the oncologist before going through for the chemo: he wanted to discuss my blood count and find out how I'd been. I wondered if I had reacted worse than most people did, whether I vomited more or less, whether other people were freaked out by the steroids. I didn't want him to think I was a baby, not able to cope.

'How have you been, Bernadette?' he asked kindly. 'I see from my notes that you were very sick after leaving the hospital last time.'

'I was,' I admitted, reluctant to complain about this too much – after all, everyone knew chemo was no picnic, and I was so grateful that I was being treated. 'But what was worse was those steroids you gave me. Do I absolutely have to have them along with the chemo? I don't think I can deal with what they do to my mind. It was scary.' I described the mind-warping hallucinations I had experienced.

'I can take you off them, to be sure,' he replied, 'but you'll certainly be sicker.'

'I'll take the sickness.' So it was agreed – no more steroids.

I had only read a few books at this point, but I had started to learn about a whole new way of dealing with cancer that no medical person had ever mentioned. I wondered whether to broach any of these alternatives with him.

'Is there anything I should be doing to help my body fight the cancer?' I asked, tentatively.

'Plenty of fresh fruit and vegetables,' he answered briskly. I nodded, but I didn't mention that I was juicing like mad already – he could have no idea just how many portions of fruit and vegetables I was consuming daily.

'I've heard that it's helpful to have a positive mental attitude.' I tried another tack.

'That's right. Chin up, you'll be fine. Right then, see you next time, Bernadette.' Clearly he wasn't going to be drawn on this point. I left hurriedly, conscious of the queue of people waiting to see him. I always felt guilty for taking up too much of his time.

Back home, the vomiting started again, and I realized that, despite my display of confidence in the oncologist's surgery, I couldn't take the sickness much longer. Now, after all, the time had come to find out more about chemotherapy, and I grabbed Jane Plant's book *Your Life in Your Hands*. It was the book that Jessica's mother had given me back when I had first been diagnosed. In it I read about a drug called Zofren which blocks the receptors in your brain which control the vomiting impulse. It wouldn't stop me feeling nauseous but it would stop the vomiting. Why hadn't I been given this? I called the chemotherapy ward and they managed to get a prescription phoned through to my local pharmacy.

That afternoon Sarah, Julie and I made our way to the chemist's. I was shaky with lack of food – again I had only managed to keep green tea down – but I was determined to get there. The pharmacist came out from behind the counter with the tablets. I knew her quite well: her mother had been Richard's head teacher.

'Mrs Bohan?' I could see from her expression that she knew exactly why I needed this drug. 'Take these every four hours on the days you feel you need to. You'll find if you purée food you may be able to keep it down.' Ugh. The idea of food made me feel ill again, but I appreciated her advice. I took the first tablet as soon as we got home. It worked, and although I could feel my body rebelling against the foreign chemicals that had been injected into it, I was no longer wracked with days of vomiting. But I didn't like the idea of taking too many drugs, particularly on top of the chemo, and I managed to reduce the Zofren to one and a half days. What more would I discover in these books? Like a contestant on *Mastermind*, cancer was my special subject and I was fast becoming something of an expert.

My weeks and months started to take on a certain shape. I would go in for chemo on a Thursday, after which I would be feeling so rotten I would need to go to bed until the Sunday. Gerard would take the Thursday and Friday off; on Saturday Sarah would be at home to help; then the whole family would be around on the

Sunday. For those first four days I would be unable to do anything at all, feeling nauseous, weak and isolated, but I would be
determined to be up again on the Monday so as to be able to look
after Julie and take her to school during the week. I would then
have nearly three weeks to get my strength back, before going for
the next chemo session on the next allotted Thursday – although
my feeling of dread would increase as the day approached.
During those precious days when I felt a little stronger, I read
and I went to all the lectures and talks I could find on health gen-
erally, and on cancer specifically. One day I'd be sitting in a
draughty church hall, on another in a smart hotel or a busy
health-food shop, and perhaps the following week in an adult
education institute. I wasn't fussy, just hungry for information,
desperate to figure it all out. And all the while I was mindful of
keeping my strength up, of not pushing my body too hard when
my white blood cell count was low, of avoiding crowds just after
the chemo sessions. The last thing I wanted was to be laid low on
any of my 'well' days, although it did happen once and I had to
go back to bed with a stomach bug. I was furious that I had been
robbed of a few good days.

'Ger,' I began, soon after the chemo had started that August, 'I
am going to have to make some changes to my diet.'

'Oh yes? Like what?' He was reading the paper and wasn't really
concentrating.

'Well, I'm going to have to cut out dairy foods for a start. I've
read in loads of places about what's in cow's milk, like hormones,
antibiotics, pesticides and chemicals. It's quite hard for our bodies

to digest, apparently. This book here is by a scientist who got breast cancer, and she points out that the incidence of breast cancer is almost non-existent in Japan where cow's milk just isn't part of their diet. She cut it out and recovered.'

'That doesn't prove it to me. Let me have a look.' He flicked through the book for a while. 'OK, well it's up to you. What about cheese – I thought you loved that?'

'I do, but I'm realizing that some of the things I have been eating might be making me sicker. I'm also worried about what milk might be doing to Julie. I know Richard and Sarah don't really drink much of it these days, but I always thought it was a healthy drink for kids and she drinks loads.'

'Fine,' he said, doing his best to be supportive. 'I think you should give it a go – what can you both have instead?' I told him about soya milk, which I had seen in health-food shops, but a few months later I switched to rice or oat milk, which is easier to digest. Like the juicing, this did not seem to be a radical change, once I got used to the taste of the new kind of milk. I missed cheese at first, but I quickly found foods to replace it with.

At the same time I had given up caffeine and alcohol, and I was starting to cut down on meat and fish. Again, they are hard for us humans to digest. I did it by putting smaller and smaller portions on my plate until it got to the point, after about six months, that I was having just a tiny square of what I by then thought of as 'cooked flesh' on my plate. I realized that it was so small it simply wasn't worth it, and I was more than happy to fill the space left by meat with more salads and raw vegetables. Of course I still cooked meat for the family, and the smell of good sausages on the barbecue would never fail to make my mouth water, just as the smell of freshly brewed coffee would make me long for a cup. Nowadays, I find the smells are enough – if I am foolish enough to try a taste, it makes me retch. I tried to get the family to make some changes along with me, but I found that was not so easy – it caused more arguments than I could handle. I didn't want them to feel I was criticizing them, nor did I want to force my new diet on them. The only thing I could do at that point was to lead by example, and like all mothers – who after all only want the best for their children – I tried to sneak in some changes without their noticing.

Making foods easier to digest was part of the secret, I was discovering, as it would free up my immune system to concentrate on getting rid of the cancer. Not only that, the mega doses of enzymes, vitamins and minerals – particularly the cancer-fighting anti-oxidants – were giving me a huge boost, and I was discovering all sorts of delicious juicing combinations now that I had invested in a new, more efficient juicer. Even Gerard and the kids were enthusiastic about the drinks I made them.

Sleeping was a problem, and I used the relaxation techniques I had learnt years before in my yoga classes – although in yoga you are supposed to stay awake, relaxed and 'mindful'. Me? I just wanted to sink into the oblivion of sleep. As soon as I got into bed I would go through the routine, and as I got better at it, so my sleep improved. Gradually I would tense and relax every single part of my body, starting with my toes and working my way up to the top of my head.

I think I became one of those irritating patients who like to think they know more than the health professionals treating them – and that was before the internet really revolutionized the lives of patients. People I see these days at my talks are incredibly well-informed and up-to-date on the latest research. One thing I used to do, for example, each time I was given the chemo, was to ask the nurse to check that she was giving me exactly the right dose. After all, I had three separate injections, and I knew all the nurses were rushed off their feet. I had also read about someone being given the wrong chemo, with disastrous results. Once, this interfering stance did pay off.

'What's that you're putting into me now?' I asked at one session that autumn.

'Hold on,' the nurse sighed, 'I'll check it for you.' I bit my lip, knowing she was annoyed. 'It's just the steroids,' she said. 'Don't worry.'

'Steroids?' I gasped. 'I'm not supposed to have them.' The nurse was incredibly apologetic. 'I'm terribly sorry, so I am. I see now it is in your notes. Most people do have the steroids as a matter of course, and I should have checked properly.'

My menopausal symptoms had started to appear – with a vengeance. I was over at my friend Lorna's house one night with a group of girlfriends, and suddenly became totally overwhelmed with heat. 'Bernie, you're flushing up,' said Mel and Helen. 'I know, and I've got palpitations too. It's this damn chemo.' I stripped my top off and soon I was sitting there in my bra. Everyone laughed at me, but for me this was the best way to cool down, and – frankly – losing my composure in front of a few good friends was the least of my problems, and these particular women were among the best of their kind. Lorna handed me a large glass of iced tap water, and I drank it gratefully. Then I remembered a leaflet I had picked up a few days earlier on the water supply – it was still in my bag and I dug it out. 'Listen to this,' I said to them, reading it out.

'Irish tap-water is fluoridated with untreated agri-fertilizer waste. Dispensed by 450 Irish water schemes to over 2.7 million consumers, it is contaminated with lead, arsenic, mercury and chromium.'

I read on, and then passed the leaflet around. It made very uncomfortable reading, yet none of us could really believe that honest-to-goodness Irish tap water could be poisoning us and our children as this leaflet seemed to suggest. There was a website and a phone number. I'd have to look into this further when I had the energy, and meanwhile I'd start buying bottled water. (I later found out that this was not a good move either.)

I did not tell my oncologist what I was doing to help myself – somehow I felt he would pooh-pooh most of it as faddy, unsubstantiated nonsense. I realized that his special area of expertise was the medical treatment of cancer and, like all medically trained doctors, he would have had less training in nutrition than the average weight-loss counsellor. This was borne out to me that October. I remember it well because it was the day he told me I was to start radiation.

Across the road from the hospital was a little health shop which I often popped into if I had some time to kill before appointments. They had a nice range of products, and ran courses on yoga, reiki and so on. I had picked up their monthly newsletter that day – as always, I read anything I could get my hands on – and was still reading it when my name was called.

'You're doing well, Bernadette,' stated my oncologist, looking at the results of that day's blood test. He could see too that I was not losing much weight, and although my hair was much thinner it wasn't falling out in chunks like some people's did. I thought this was because of the digestive enzymes and the juicing – I was retaining many more of the nutrients my body needed than I otherwise would have been able to do. But I said nothing. 'I think we can start you on the radiation a week on Monday. You'll be in every weekday for five weeks, and of course the chemo will still continue every third Thursday.'

'Is there anything I should know before I start?' I ventured to ask.

'Not really. Your appointments will be in the mornings, so if I were you I'd plan to give yourself plenty of rest afterwards. You'll be feeling quite tired.' Jesus, if he warned me that I'd be tired that meant I'd be totally bloody exhausted.

I inadvertently left the newsletter on my chair as I got up to leave. He seized it and waved it scornfully at me, reading out the headline: *Shock News: Anti-perspirants and deodorants may cause cancer.* 'Christ Almighty, some of us have to get PhDs before we can advise people suffering from cancer and this guy just sets himself up over the road. None of this is proven.' I knew he was wrong, but did not have the facts at my fingertips – as I do now.

I was very nervous when I went in for the first radiation session, not knowing what to expect. Nurse Angie tattooed some tiny black marks around my breast, pinpointing the area where the radiation would be applied. She showed me where to lie, directly underneath the huge machine, and then she left me alone in the room. 'Don't move,' she warned. Dear God, I thought, how on earth do they get children to lie still for this? The machine was lowered by an invisible operator until it was a few centimetres above me. The actual radiation itself lasted for a few minutes and at first I felt nothing. Then, after a few days of this, I saw I had what looked like sunburn. A week later I was very, very burnt – and I wasn't even half-way through the treatment. I would go round the house with a soft T-shirt on, no bra underneath. One Sunday lunch I was so sore I said to Richard, 'Would you mind if I took my shirt off? It's so painful; the chafing of the material is agony.'

'Oh Mum, no!'

'Please, please,' I begged him. 'At least let me unbutton it. You don't have to look.'

'OK, but you can pay for the therapy later,' he grumbled. Fair enough, I realize now as I write this: at eighteen you don't really need to get an eyeful of your mum's breasts. But at that point – sick with the chemo, worn out by the radiation – I was too sore to worry about his sensibilities.

Some people get sick with radiation. It didn't hit me that way, but the oncologist was right about the tiredness: it totally floored me. It sapped every last ounce of energy. Each morning I'd drop Julie off at school if I had enough time before my appointment, or if not, Sarah would take her in. There would always be a wait of around half an hour, then with luck I'd be home by around 11am. I'd go straight to bed and set the alarm for 1.00pm, so I could wake and go to fetch Julie at 1.30. I knew I couldn't opt out of her life for five weeks – it was important for us both that I carried on as best as I could. At least I had no trouble sleeping during the radiation.

'Mama, are we going trick or treating next week?' asked Julie one morning. My heart sank – of course she'd want to do this, as it was something we always did together. There aren't many kids down our way, but the neighbours always laugh at what Julie and I turn up wearing, and make sure they have a little treat for her. I was determined that she wasn't going to miss out that year, so I got us both kitted out as Morticia and Wednesday Addams. As I checked my thin, wasted reflection in the hall mirror before we left, Julie clutching her goodie bag, I thought ruefully that I would have made quite a realistic ghost.

I started to learn visualization techniques, so that when I was lying under that terrible machine I could imagine myself else-where. Starting with my relaxation exercise, I would end by taking myself to a cool green forest where I would hear birdsong and the rushing of waterfalls. Inside my head I had my own private paradise: it was simple, but it did help me cope with the fear and the worry, and it made me feel that I had some control over what was being done to me. I felt that this, at that point, would help me more than prayer.

There were times during the treatment, particularly when I had the radiation and chemo simultaneously, that I felt like giving in. It was so hard, I felt so low and worn out, I looked wretched, a useless shell of a person. I was learning to support myself physically – a process I now think of as 'changing over' – but mentally I felt I was falling apart. Gerard and the kids were fantastic throughout, and I used to lie in bed listening to their noise and chatter downstairs and wish more than anything that I could be down there with them. I was so grateful, too, for the support of friends and neighbours who were always dropping round or calling to find out if there was anything they could get for me, or anywhere they could drive me to. Throughout that year I was constantly being reminded of how much women help each other in times of need: they just get stuck in and do whatever it takes. In particular, Patricia, Grace and Sharon were unwavering and totally unselfish in their help and I don't know if I could have got through it without them.

Patricia lives some way from my house, in a village just outside a town called Swords. It's real country out there – she grows her own vegetables and has a cow and a horse. I bumped into her at the supermarket just after I had been diagnosed the second time.

'I don't suppose you know anywhere I can find organic fruit and vegetables?' I asked her, thinking that with her countryside connections she might well know. I was starting to worry that the pesticides and fertilizer residues in 'normal' fruit and veg would be getting through to me in higher doses because of juicing. She didn't – in those days (only five years ago!) it was hard to find organic produce – but as soon as she realized I was sick she promised to help me. The supplier we found was quite a drive away, so Patricia would go shopping for me on the days I was laid low with chemo, bringing me all the supplies I needed for my juicer.

Grace was with me for several of my appointments, and often took me to the hospital when I was too weak to drive myself. I don't know how she managed to keep me smiling, but she did. What we went through together cemented what was already a good friendship. Sharon is my sister-in-law, married to Ger's brother Paul. These days I don't see her much, but that year she was there, almost miraculously, whenever I needed her. She would appear on the Saturdays after my chemo and just get stuck in to whatever needed to be done – she walked the dog, cleaned the bathrooms, did the shopping, and – best of all – played with Julie. Sometimes she would go home looking like a dog's dinner, with her hair all over the place after Julie had been playing hairdressers with her; other times she would drive off with her face painted with wild squiggles and zigzags. She would just shrug her shoulders and grin. When I talk to her on the phone I always end by saying, 'I love you.' She was embarrassed at first, but now she's used to it and tells me she loves me too. She is eight years younger than me, but our birthdays are on the same day, and I always add her name to my cake.

It may sound corny, but I have learnt that you have to take the opportunities to tell people you love them. Life is precarious, and we have a choice as to how we deal with the knowledge that people we care about may not be here next year, next month, or even tomorrow. I believe it is up to us to give out as much love as we can. During my illness I decided never to be one of those people who say uselessly, 'But I never told him how much I loved him.' I had made this mistake with my father, and I regretted it bitterly.

Despite all this help and support with which I was surrounded, one terrible day I was on my own in the house when Richard walked through the door. He had been in an accident. His face was white, and he seemed to be having difficulty breathing. I was on the sofa recovering from the morning's radiation – having struggled to get there in the first place – and quite unable to get up. I gave a little cry when I saw him. 'What on earth has happened?'

'Mum. I'm OK, don't fuss, but we drove into the back of a car.'

'What? How?'

'The car in front crashed into another car, and we couldn't stop in time. I was in the back, but I'd only just got in and was taking off my jacket before buckling my seatbelt. So I was thrown forwards.'

'Where does it hurt?'

'My chest. And my back is sore.' Jesus, I thought. He might have broken a rib, or done some damage to his spine or neck. I had to get him to hospital, but how? I hated the cancer more than ever then, for preventing me from taking proper care of my child. I knew, of course, that Gerard would have come immediately, or anyone I chose to call. But I felt it was my job to go with him, and I wept as I saw him get into the back of a taxi, cursing this feeling of utter helplessness.

Richard was fine, as it turned out, but a few days later I received a call from Aquinas. 'Mum's had another stroke.'

'Oh no, no more.' I couldn't deal with this – yet another blow to deal with when I was already on my knees.

'The doctors don't think she'll make it this time. I've been told to get hold of all the family.' I perked up a little: that meant I'd be seeing Jimmy, my favourite brother. He lived in England, and my world had collapsed when, in his early twenties, he had moved away from home. I called him to tell him about the summons to the hospital.

'Bernie, how are you doing? Are you bearing up?' He knew I was sick – my sisters had told him when I'd got the diagnosis.

'What about Gerard and the kids, are they OK?' I told him how things were, and I broke the news about our mother. 'Listen,' he said. 'She's at the end of her life. You're only in the middle of yours. I can't wait to see you.'

'I look like shit,' I said.

It was her 89th birthday the following week, and we all congregated in her hospital room, taking photos, believing this was the last we would see of our dear little mum. Bless her, her mind had gone, and she didn't really know who we were, although I felt she knew at some level that her time was limited. How I longed to put my arms around her and tell her all my problems like I used to do as a child. I thought of Marti Caine, who had suffered greatly with cancer a few years earlier. (I had followed her progress, which sadly was downhill, with great interest and empathy, as you do when high-profile public figures are going through a similar experience to your own.) Something she said had stuck in my mind. That her mother, who had many failings later in life, gave her enough love in her first seven years to enable her to withstand all the hard knocks life was to deal her. This is how I felt about my own mother, and as I stroked her pale cheek I reflected that it was probably a good thing that she would never know that I, her baby, had cancer. I sat and put my arms around her, trying to comfort her and draw what strength I could from her frail body. I remembered how, as a child, we used to sit cosily together, before the big ones got back from school, in front of *Watch with Mother*. She would be in her pinny and there would always be a smell of baking in the house. If I shut my eyes I could almost imagine the smell of her scones and brown bread.

Gerard was talking to Jimmy, Aquinas, and her husband Pat, and Sarah and Julie were in a corner with Deirdre, Terence and Frank. Richard was next to me, and I knew how shaken he was to see someone so near death – she looked even worse than I did, and that was saying something. As I sat hugging her, lost in my own memories, he put an arm around me, saying quietly, 'It's all right, Mum, it's all right.' The poor lad could see I needed my own mother, and in his inarticulate way he was doing his best to show me that he could be my support, now that she no longer could be. Eventually he led me out, but I so wanted to stay with her. I had spent days by my father's bedside when he was dying but I never said goodbye to him and I hadn't been with him when he died. I did not want to leave my mother by herself now.

The fact that, a week later, my mother was sitting up in bed as if nothing had happened did not take away the sharp sense that, although I was going through my own private hell, life – and death – was still going on around me. I couldn't put it on hold and ask it to wait until I was feeling more able to deal with it. And in some ways I did not want to: one strange upside to all this, I noticed, was that my senses were heightened. Food tasted of itself once more – or was it my new diet? Smells were richer and stronger, landscapes more beautiful, people kinder, music more evocative, more sensual … and Ger's touch, or the feel of Julie's hand in mine, was like I had never felt before. In the middle of all the horror I was discovering how precious life was. Suddenly I became highly observant, and had a new, acute appreciation of my world. It was a primal instinct, a visceral desire to keep going. This, I realized, was a privilege. A privilege offered only to those living on the edge.

And still I forced myself to go out to lectures and talks, although sometimes Gerard would try to make me stay at home and rest. 'These people know what I need to know,' I would insist. 'I must go.' It was on the days that I was confined to bed, however, that I really learnt the most, as I could do nothing else. I must admit that I was confused by some of what I was reading. In one place I would read of certain vitamins that were essential; then one speaker would say that the therapeutic amounts of vitamins recommended by some people were toxic. I was unsure about cooking vegetables too: steaming had been my preferred way of cooking, believing that it preserved the goodness; then I read that key nutrients were destroyed by cooking at a temperature greater than 45 degrees. Then at one lecture I heard about sprouting – a way of growing vegetable seeds into sprouts that contain fifty to a hundred times more nutrients than the grown vegetable. This was worth getting out of bed for! It didn't involve the confusing field of vitamins, and they could be eaten raw. I was determined to find out more, and start as soon as possible. What was more, during the course of my six months of chemotherapy, and beyond, I met some of the best-known names in the health field and pumped them for information.

It was almost Christmas, and I was due to go in for my penultimate chemotherapy session just before the day itself. I couldn't bear to think that Julie's Christmas would be ruined by my being sick, and I asked the oncologist if there was any way he could delay it.

'Sure we can, a week won't make any difference at this stage. There are always several operatives off that week anyway.' I was so pleased, and so grateful – having four weeks rather than only three in between bouts was heaven, and we had a lovely family Christmas. Gerard was in high spirits throughout the holiday, and said to me on several occasions, 'Isn't it great – only two more to go!' That was not how I felt at all. I knew I would dread it right to the end – like climbing a mountain, to others it looks as if you are nearly there; for me the final peak was the worst, and seemed almost insurmountable. My immune system was at its lowest point, and despite all my efforts to keep myself as healthy as I could, I knew I was almost at breaking point. I couldn't wait for the year 2000 to be behind me.

When it was eventually all over, the oncologist said to me gently, 'Those last two sessions were very tough on you, weren't they?' I nodded, and lay still as he examined me. What was supposed to happen now, I wondered? Was I free to go home and get on with my life? I think he read my expression.

'Well now, the chemo and radiotherapy should have removed all cancerous cells. Your immune system will hopefully repair itself. Don't worry, I'll keep a close eye on you. I got you out of it the first time, and I've got you out of it a second time! Come back every three months for a check-up.'

As I left the hospital I noticed the first few snowdrops of spring pushing their way through the hard earth. I was bowed, but not broken. The tumour was gone, and I had only lost half a stone in weight. My hair was starting to thicken, and – astonishingly – my arthritis in my right hand and shoulder seemed to have disappeared. I also found I no longer needed my reading glasses. I thought about the few simple changes I had made to my lifestyle, and realized there was no turning back now.

'So, are you going to give up this health kick now you're through the treatment?' said Ger a few days after the final session of chemo.

'You must be joking,' I laughed. 'There's no way I am ever going to revisit that hell again – not if I have anything to do with it.'

And I did have something to do with it. Now, more than ever, I understood that my future was in my own hands.

Chapter Seventeen

Breaking Through

J ust as stress sets off a kind of vicious circle in which your anxieties and fears stop you from looking after yourself properly, which in turn leads to illness and disease within the body, so I found that once I turned the corner into a healthy way of life, I started to feel the benefits. I had more energy than I had had for years, which in turn motivated me to look after my body much more effectively. Naturally, it helped enormously that the treatment was over, but I knew that I would not be regarded as totally 'cured' for many years yet. The simple but dramatic changes I had made to my way of life – which had started as a stark choice between eating and drinking as I used to, or filling my shopping trolley with different items – were now no longer a choice. It was simply the way I was going to keep myself well.

Malahide is a small town, and at that time we had lived there for sixteen years, so we knew a fair few people – having three children at two different schools widens your circle of acquaintances like nothing else! During my illness, though, the number of people I saw regularly had contracted to some close girlfriends, a few local neighbours and my family. It wasn't until the spring of 2001 that life returned to normal and my health and spirits began to improve, and I was able to get out a bit more often.

'Bernadette Bohan?' came a cry from behind me as I window-shopped along the local high street one crisp March morning. 'Is that really you?' I turned to see a woman with whom I'd made some costumes for a school play some years earlier.

'Hello,' I said warmly, trying to remember her name. 'How are you doing?'

'Oh, I'm fine, back at work now that Sean is in full-time school. How are your three kids?' I told her what they were all doing, and took a few steps along the pavement as if to carry on with my shopping, but she carried on talking as if there was something she had to say.

'You look well, though, Bernadette. I, er, I hope you don't mind me asking, but, um, I heard you have been very ill.'

'That's right. Breast cancer.'

'Didn't you have cancer that other time?' I nodded. 'You've had it twice?'

'Yeah, that's right,' I smiled.

'How come you are looking so good?' There. She'd said it. I guessed from her face that when she'd heard that I had had cancer a second time she'd assumed that I had either already died or must be on my way out. A fair assumption, I reasoned.

'I started finding out about ways to beat cancer through eating more healthily. I've discovered some amazing things. Now I drink massive quantities of organic vegetable juice, I drink lots of clean water, I grow my own sprouts, I take digestive enzymes and probiotics and –'

'Brussels sprouts?' she interrupted.

'No, I have little jars in my kitchen where I grow all kinds of seeds – alfalfa, fenugreek, broccoli – and when they have sprouted a few shoots I eat them with salads or in a sandwich. They're powerhouses of nutrients – you wouldn't believe what they contain.'

We carried on chatting while we walked back up the street, and she eventually told me that her husband had prostate cancer. Ah, I thought, that explained her fierce interest in my recovery. Then I suddenly realized we were near my house. 'Come in, why don't you? I'll show you my juicer and how I do the sprouting.'

She spent two hours with me that day, and returned a few days later to find out more. That time she brought a friend with her whose daughter had just been diagnosed with breast cancer. A week later the daughter herself came: a pretty, dark girl in her twenties. I could see she was frightened, and desperate for help. She had that same hunger for information and knowledge that I had felt myself not so very long ago. 'I want to get on your programme,' she said. 'Tell me exactly what to do.' That shocked me. I had not thought of what I had been doing as a plan, or a programme, it was just a few things I did, based on what I thought was some very compelling evidence.

'My goodness!' I exclaimed, a little embarrassed. 'I'm not suggesting this is a programme you can follow, but I can show you a few simple things that will have a huge impact on your health.'

'I'd really appreciate that, if it's not too much trouble.' Too much trouble? This was my special subject, and I loved nothing more than climbing up on my soapbox.

'OK. The first thing you need to understand is that cancer is caused by deficiency and toxicity. Your job is to maintain a powerful immune system to help you fight the disease. You can do this by removing some known carcinogens from your environment, and by adding certain things to your diet – delicious things, I might add – which will give your body massive doses of the anti-oxidant vitamins and certain minerals and enzymes that it needs for recovery.'

'What about chemotherapy, and radiotherapy, and should I have a mastectomy, and what about manual lymph drainage?' the questions tumbled forth.

'I cannot advise you on any of that; I'm not a medical person, although I can tell you about my own experience. You must make your own decisions, but educate yourself so that you can make an informed decision. What I can show you are the extra things you can do to enhance your chances of survival.' And so I would go on, and the hours would pass. This would happen several times a week, and my first few 'students' would leave, gratefully clutching handfuls of scribbled notes.

I'm a sociable, chatty person, and everywhere I went I would talk to people, and I would tell them what I was doing. My new diet seemed to be so effective, and I was so excited to be feeling well and to feel I actually had a future ahead of me, that I became something of an evangelist. The more I talked about it, the more people would contact me to ask if I could explain what to do about cleaning up their water, and which toiletries didn't have damaging chemicals in them, or where to find the best organic products. I was receiving two or three phone calls per day from people suffering not just from cancer, but from arthritis, eczema, ME, irritable bowel syndrome, and many other ailments. And what was even more interesting, perhaps, was that most people who contacted me were fit and well – and wanted to stay that way.

'How long is this going to go on for?' asked Gerard grumpily one evening, as our dinner was interrupted by yet another telephone call.

'Sorry, won't be long,' I said breezily as I rushed off to take the call.

'I meant how long are you going to be acting as unofficial health adviser to the entire population of Dublin?' he said when I returned.

'Yeah,' chimed in the others. 'It's getting a bit much. The house isn't our own any more.'

It was true. It wasn't just phone calls: most days I was in the kitchen with two or more people, usually strangers, trying out juicing combinations, showing them which supplements were worth buying, giving them information about the dangers of fluoride … sometimes I did not have much time to prepare the family's evening meal, and quiet evenings with Gerard were often derailed by the telephone. And, if I admitted it, I was tired out as well.

'I'm sorry, I realize it's hard on all of you. Perhaps I ought to group people into proper classes and hold them at regular times, and only speak to people on the phone at certain times.'

'Or perhaps you could stop altogether?' they said.

'I can't, this is too important. I have information that could help these people. I can't not tell them what I know.'

'I think it was your determination and drive to live that saved you. You were completely focussed on finding ways to help your-self, and it was that which pulled you through. Not this faddy diet thing.' My heart sank. This was Gerard, my Mr Wonderful. If he didn't believe in my diet, who would?

'You would think like me if you had read all the evidence,' I insisted. 'And look at me – surely you are pleased I have helped myself become well again? Don't forget how I used to moan about my arthritis. And only last week my dentist said he couldn't believe the improvement in my gums and teeth!'

'Of course I am pleased, but evidence?' he snorted. 'Are you telling me that there is a cure for cancer out there and your oncologist isn't telling you about it? Don't be daft.'

'You know what doctors are like   they want to have everything proven and tested and re-tested in double-blind trials like drugs are. Who's going to invest millions of pounds in doing those kinds of trials on this stuff? I think it's just common sense.'

'Well, all I know is, you can't continue with it for ever.'

'Why not?'

'Well, surely it's hard cooking separate meals for the rest of us. All that shopping for organic fruit, and those supplements you're taking. And as for not drinking milk – where do you think you're going to get your calcium from? Thin air? You're cured, aren't you? Can't you just accept that, and move on?' Then he let slip the real reason for his hostility. 'And it's so difficult for everyone else. You make us feel as if we're being really unhealthy.'

I had had a similar reaction from my sisters and friends, who assumed that now the cancer had apparently gone I would give up what they saw as a flaky, alternative lifestyle. People who were incredibly supportive while I had cancer and was going through the treatment suddenly developed a distinctly frosty approach, or merely dismissed what I was saying. They wanted the old me back, and I understood. It was threatening to them that I was choosing a new path: deep down they probably suspected that I was on to something, but they were simply not ready to do it themselves. I felt as if I was living a double life – admired by some, opposed by others. I had gone from being the object of everyone's sympathy to someone who was being praised and sought out by sick people; but criticized, almost shunned, by those I loved best. It felt oddly schizophrenic. My own family was still the worst. I had another shot at getting them onto a more healthy diet, but failed miserably. They loved some of the juices, but they wouldn't give up their pizzas, steaks and biscuits. 'What if you get sick?' I asked Gerard once. 'I'll wait until I get ill,' he retorted. 'Until then, I'll take my chances.'

Even Richard thought I was turning into a hippie, by which he meant that I was frequenting organic markets and health-food stores rather too much. He and Sarah refused to give up the foods I told them were harming them, or follow much of my new diet although I tried so hard to explain the benefits. 'We're young; we don't care!' was what they said. Of course – they felt immortal. I remembered that feeling. It was different with Julie: she was young enough to accept changes to her diet without complaining, and hardly noticed the switch from cow's milk to soya. The only problems I had with her were when the bigger ones tried to undermine what I was doing. 'What's that, Julie?' they would say. 'What's she giving you now?' and the little thing would be torn between wanting to do as I asked her and wanting to please her big brother and sister. Gerard, too, didn't want her to be different from other kids and miss out on ice creams and other 'treats'. I know the dangers that lurk in sugar, and I know the attraction it holds for children – as the baby of the family I was always first in line for any treats, and would be given a spoon of sugar if there was nothing else. It is still a struggle to keep Julie on the straight and narrow, but I comfort myself with the thought that if I have done nothing else, at least my family has clean water and they drink more freshly juiced fruit and vegetables than most people. There is an old Irish saying: *you can pull with a string but you can't push with it.* I often used to say to them in frustration, 'You're old enough to make your own choices. At least I know I have done my duty and told you the facts.' As for old sweet-tooth Gerard, I know he'd be as fat as a fool by now if I hadn't had some impact on his diet.

One afternoon Sarah asked me for a lift into the village, a five minutes' walk away. I was busy juicing. 'No,' I said. 'You've a fine pair of legs on you – the walk will do you good.'

'Oh, for God's sake! All you think about these days is yourself,' she huffed. That wasn't quite true, but I had to acknowledge that I was determined to stay focussed on my new 'programme', and I had moved on from the days when my main motivation was to keep myself alive for my children. Now I was more mature, and I wanted to live for myself as well. And I was getting a real buzz out of helping other people.

Then one day I received a letter (in fact, the first of hundreds) which made it all worth it, and made me realize I had no option but to continue, whatever the cost. I include some of it here:

Dear Bernadette

What a fortuitous day 8 April was, the day I met my new friend Vera who gave me your name and number. I didn't know it then, but it was the day the sun shone on my future.

As soon as I heard I had Hodgkin's disease I was determined to research a more holistic way of living so I could make some positive health changes. I was looking for something to address my whole system, not just my lymphomas.

I must tell you how touched I was that you immediately accommodated me on your current class, and gave me some very sound advice to be getting on with … I thoroughly enjoyed your talks and they served as a wonderful one-stop shop for information on nutritional therapy and other lifestyle changes that made perfect sense. Although I wasn't new to the benefits of juicing and some of the other ideas, I was very enlightened by the 'green' healing juices and wheatgrass. I was consistently impressed by how well researched you were.

I am very excited to have learned this stuff whilst my family is still young, so we can treat my illness as a great opportunity to address our food habits. Everybody now gets excited here when the juices appear and a dark green 'kale' moustache is a common sight in our house!

Finally, I was really moved when you wouldn't accept any money from me for the course. Thank you for your kindness. I met two other new friends there also, and they have continued to support me throughout my chemotherapy treatment. It has opened up a whole new world of knowledge and friendship.

I will keep in touch with you. Many, many thanks again.

Lena McMyler

I decided to confine the classes I was giving to one day of the week: Mondays. In the mornings I would teach one group, and in the evenings another. The entire course would last four weeks, and each class was supposed to last one hour, but often ran over. Some of these people had travelled long distances to see me, and many of them had painful stories to share. We started with juicing, moved on to food, clean water, supplements and personal-care products. I took care not to make any of it daunting, just concentrating on the few simple things that people could do in their own homes. Many of them were overwhelmed with the amount of conflicting, confusing information out there. They didn't want to be told that there were twenty-seven thousand different things they could do to improve their health; they wanted the four or five main ideas. I discovered that these few simple changes that were so alienating for my friends and family were a lifeline for those people who had, as I had done, looked into the abyss.

And so it continued. I did try my best to fit my new activities around my family's needs, and as more and more people came to me I found I needed to start planning, booking classes up to three months ahead. It had never been difficult for me to teach people in my kitchen, but the more practice I had at explaining things, the more I felt I was helping them. I tried to be light-hearted, to have a bit of craic and to be practical too. I knew these were frightened people who were being bombarded with too much information from all sides – from their doctors, from friends, from their own reading – and I knew from my own experience how hard it was to see a way through. I wanted to offer them hope; to show them that in the midst of their suffering and fear there could be a ray of light. And at the same time I was developing a new sense of purpose – 'spreading the word' was now my mission. I felt I had to reach more people.

So when I was approached one day about speaking at a local school, I knew I ought to do it. Here was an opportunity to tell more people about what they could do to help themselves, whether they were sick or well. But my initial reaction was one of apprehension. I had never in my life stood up and spoken in front of an audience before. 'How many people will be there?' I asked the organizer, playing for time.

'We don't know yet, but there is room for around a hundred people in the hall. The other speakers include a dentist, a doctor and a pharmacist.'

'But those are all professional people,' I said, aware of a new worm of fear wriggling in my stomach. 'I'm just an ordinary person. I don't have any qualifications to speak.'

'Well, Mrs Bohan, all I can say is I keep hearing your name. You have survived cancer, and you teach people about all kinds of health topics. It seems to me that you have something to say that people want to hear.' So I agreed.

I spent hours preparing my little talk, rehearsing in front of Gerard and the kids. I was nervous, but excited. Ger came with me to the talk, and as we entered the school hall I realized that in the audience were many of the people who sent their kids to school with mine. I was one of them, but here I was about to get up and tell them what to do! I sat in the front, listening to the other talks. The doctor dithered on about vaccinations, the dental nurse was quite interesting about children's lunchboxes, and the pharmacist told people what to do about head lice – very helpful for that audience, I reflected. Then it was my turn. I stood up, my legs trembling with anxiety.

'Ladies and Gentlemen,' I began. 'Those of you here who know me will know that I am no doctor, scientist or health guru. I am a mother of three kids, and in the course of my life I have developed cancer twice. Sixteen years ago it was in my lymph system, and when I recovered I followed what I thought was a healthy-enough lifestyle: a bowl of muesli, two pieces of fruit and some steamed veggies. The second time was little more than eighteen months ago, and this time I decided to educate myself. I was astounded by what I discovered and I started to make a few simple changes to the way I lived my life. Everyone has their own way of dealing with something like cancer. I'm not saying mine is the only way, or that it is the best way, and I'm not promising that it will save lives, but it has worked for me. I feel and look better than I have done in years, my arthritis has disappeared and eyesight has improved, and my only regret is that I did not change over to a healthier lifestyle years ago. Tonight I am going to tell you about one element of your diet that is crucially important – whether you are sick or well. Essential fats.' I had my sheaf of notes, but suddenly I realized I did not need them. As I warmed to my subject, I saw people leaning forward with interest, nodding, whispering to their neighbours, and making notes. Making notes! When I eventually finished, the applause went on for some time. The other speakers drifted off home, and an hour later I was still surrounded by eager people asking questions and begging for more information.

'I'm so proud of you,' said Ger as we climbed into bed that night. 'You have a real gift for communication – and I never realized!' I glowed with pleasure, still high from my success and so pleased that Gerard was acknowledging my efforts. 'No, really,' he went on, 'you were calm and funny, and really held their attention. I could see them listening hard. And I have to say, you're a great advert for this "system" of yours. You've never looked better.' This was praise indeed, and I knew that Gerard was now back as my biggest supporter.

I gave several more lectures in hotels, health centres and church halls, and each time I got a little better at delivering my talks, although I was always frightened beforehand. The audiences were fairly small, yet all the time I could feel that demand was escalating for whatever it was that I was offering, and there grew a germ of an idea in the back of my mind. At first I hardly dared admit the idea to myself, let alone discuss it with Gerard. The annual 'Your Health' show was coming up. It was held in Dublin's RDS. They expected around six thousand visitors every day for three days, and anyone who was anyone in the increasingly large health field had a stand at the show, and – this was what was exercising my mind – there was a strong programme of lectures from authors, nutritionists and other health practitioners. It would be nearly three years since I had finished the chemo; I had amassed a huge amount of information, I had taught many people in my own home and given talks to hundreds more. What was more, I was living proof that what I was advocating had a hugely positive effect on my own health. Did I dare offer myself as a speaker?

'What do you reckon, Ger?' I asked him after dinner one evening, having outlined my plan.

'Go for it, Bernie, I'm with you all the way.'

'Do you think I can do it?'

'I know you can do it.'

'I'm not so sure. I mean, I'm just an ordinary woman who's survived cancer – for now.'

'Come off it, you're much more than that. Lots of people have cancer, and some people survive. But you've got something to tell people that you believe will really help them. You're willing to stand up and be counted, and you're helping others. How many people can say that about themselves?'

I was still unsure, but a few days later I received a letter from someone who had been at one of my talks. It read: **I was sitting at the back of your lecture last week. I never heard a word you said, but just to look at you and to know that you are still alive was enough.** She had cancer, and I knew exactly how she felt: so many times I had been to lectures by scientists and nutritionists and wondered how they could possibly understand what they were talking about if they had never been in my position. It was that letter that clinched it for me. If I could help just one single person, it would be worth it. So I wrote to the organizers of 'Your Health', putting myself forward as a speaker.

I heard back within a few weeks. To my astonishment I was offered three slots, one on each day of the show. I was to talk at 3pm, a good time, but I would be competing against some famous speakers and writers. I was full of excitement, but horrified at my recklessness. How on earth was I going to do this? Who did I think I was?

But there was no going back now: this was the breakthrough I had waited for.

Chapter Eighteen

Spreading the Word

As the day of the health show approached, the sick feeling in the pit of my stomach got worse every time I thought about it. How time had dragged during my months of illness, and how quickly it seemed to be rushing by now! If only I had not put myself forward, I groaned to myself. And if only I hadn't been accepted. How on earth could I have had the gall to imagine I could stand up as a speaker alongside those famous names? Who did I think I was to tell people how to change their lives? It was ridiculous; I would have to get out of it somehow. I racked my brains for excuses. Perhaps I could claim urgent family business? I was a rotten liar, I'd never sound convincing. Or could I just phone and say I had changed my mind? That would work, but it sounded cowardly. And as for writing the speech itself, I kept putting it off, hoping that the whole thing would go away.

After twenty-odd years of marriage I find that Ger is pretty astute when it comes to picking up my moods. Although I hadn't said anything to him, he knew exactly what was bothering me.

'Need any help with your talk?' he asked casually one evening after dinner. 'It's coming up pretty soon isn't it?' I guess that was the opening I had subconsciously been waiting for, because out tumbled all my fears and worries. The strange thing was that as I told him what had been on my mind it all sounded so silly. He put his arms around me and laughed.

'Bernie, don't be daft,' he said. 'I know you can do it, and you know you can do it. You've every bit as much right to stand up and talk to a room full of people as these so-called famous names. Look at you! You say you're just an ordinary woman, but if I was going to one of these talks that is just the kind of person I'd want to hear speak. Someone who has been through something like cancer twice, and come through the other side. You have done your research – it's not as if you've made this stuff up. And you don't just spout theories, you really practise what you preach. In fact, you'll be preaching what you've practised!' And so he went on, knocking down every one of my objections until I was almost convinced I would be all right.

'I promise you, you'll go down a storm,' he said finally. 'I've heard you talk many times. You always come across well – you're confident, warm, and you make difficult ideas easy to understand. Come on now, let's start planning it.'

That night I covered the kitchen table with the notes I had made for previous talks. They ranged across all sorts of subjects: juicing, sprouting, clean water, supplements, cancer-fighting foods. I wondered whether to expand on one particular area or cobble together a mish-mash of all of them.

'What is it you want to tell people?' asked Ger. 'Put it in a nut-shell for me.' I thought for a moment.

'I suppose it is my belief that you don't have to change a lot of things about your lifestyle to make a huge difference to your own health and chances of fighting illness, and that these few things are quite simple when you know how.'

'So you are telling people that if they can just manage to change a little, it will help them a great deal.'

'Yes, that's it.' Suddenly it clicked. 'I've got it! Change a little – it helps a lot. What a great title!' I sat down and immediately started drafting my talk. I would bring in something from *all* the lectures and classes I had given – this was my big opportunity to get my simple message across and I wasn't going to mess it up.

Ger has done a bit of public speaking in the course of his business life, and he helped me structure the speech. I practised in front of him and the children – they were so good really, listening to me when they wanted to be off doing other things – until I knew it off by heart. I then made brief notes on cards to spark my memory. Again I practised until I was word perfect. I was still nervous, but at least I knew now what I was going to say.

The big day finally arrived, and I was shaking with nerves all the way to the RDS exhibition centre in Dublin, suffering from the nausea that comes from too much adrenalin. On a notice board outside the main hall I saw a poster listing that day's talks: Patrick Holford was talking on Fatigue, Anxiety, Insomnia and

Depression; Dr Gillian McKeith on Boosting Immunity. These two coincided directly with my talk, and sounded to me like they would draw big crowds. There were other talks that I thought I might try to go to later if I got the chance: one on Digestive Problems, another on Nutrition for the Menopause and one on Managing Arthritis. I counted around twenty speakers each day, split between five lecture rooms. This was a big deal, and I was terrified. Calm down, I told myself, attempting to do my relaxation exercise then and there.

I had an hour or so to kill before my slot, so I wandered around the show marvelling at the number of different health products on offer. I watched some people having reiki massages, saw others having their auras photographed and still others lying with moxibustion candles in their ears. Some of what I saw seemed pretty weird, and I was glad I did not have to explain anything more difficult than simple nutritional facts.

Suddenly I heard an announcement over the loudspeaker system: *Bernadette Bohan's talk CHANGE A LITTLE – IT HELPS A LOT starts in ten minutes in lecture room 4.* This was it – and in an hour it would all be over. I had asked for a small room, not being confident of getting much of an audience, and breathed a sigh of relief on that first day when I saw about thirty-five people dotted around the room waiting for me. I stood behind the table at the top of the room, swallowed hard, and tried to pretend this was just another talk in a school hall. 'You are all very welcome,' I began. 'I am going to talk to you about preventing cancer.' As usual, once I had started I just got on with it, and found I even enjoyed it. I knew my material so well I was even able to throw in a few jokes. So I got through it, and was pleased with the applause and the genuinely interested questions afterwards. If I can just get through two more days like this, I thought, I'll be doing fine. Then I can retreat to my life of relative obscurity, giving my little classes, and I won't venture out to something like this again.

The next day the number had doubled in my little room. I saw that there were a few people from the previous day's talk back again. That gave me a boost, and it was nice to be able to smile at a few friendly faces while giving my talk. Again, I felt it went down well and people were terribly kind and complimentary afterwards. Several people commented on how 'do-able' it all was. 'Of course it is,' I said. 'I had an eighteen-year-old going through exams, a sixteen-year-old going through puberty and a five-year-old starting school – and I was going through chemotherapy and radiotherapy at the same time. If I can do it, anyone can!'

I was just patting myself on the back for getting through it a second time, when a smartly dressed man who had been at the back of the room approached me. 'You have given me so much hope,' was all he said. He had tears in his eyes. It was for people like him that I was putting myself through this, I realized. How I wished I could tell my mother what I was doing.

'I think you'll need a larger room tomorrow,' said one of the organizers as I was packing up my things. 'Oh no,' I begged him. 'This one will do just fine.' 'Well, all right,' he agreed, 'but I'll bring in more chairs just in case.'

Over breakfast the next day I announced to the family: 'I think I'll be confident enough today to come out from behind that table. It's been much easier than I thought, and people are so receptive.' But later on that day when I breezed up the stairs to deliver my talk I had to edge my way through a crowd of people blocking the corridor. My heart sank – I'd only be getting a few people today if there was another popular speaker. Never mind, I'd be finished soon, no harm done.

'Who are you all queuing for?' I asked one elderly lady.

'Bernadette Bohan,' came the astonishing reply. And sure enough, there was my room with a long line of people waiting to go in. I squeezed through the door to find a packed room with people crushed into the aisles on extra chairs, and many sitting on the window sills. Several people stood at the back, and I heard later that they had to turn people away. There was a rustle of excitement as I made my way to the front of the room. I could forget about the table, there was hardly any space for me to move. All eyes were on me. 'Jesus, Mary Mother of God,' I muttered. 'Make me do this right for them.' The room fell silent as I started to speak. I now felt I knew exactly what to say, and how to say it; I believed they were listening and that what I was saying made sense.

'These few do-able changes will go a long way to improving your health.' I was coming to the end of my talk. 'Good health is about taking responsibility for yourself and informing and educating ourselves on what we put in our mouths and use on our bodies. But I hope what I have told you today will inspire you to start to make some of these simple changes in your own life. It's not rocket science, and you can do it in your own kitchen.'

The applause was deafening, and many people rushed up to see me afterwards. So many people wanted to talk to me, to ask me specific questions about what they should do for themselves or their loved ones, and to know where they could find out more. Their need for information and reassurance was palpable – each person clearly had an urgent desire for help – and I knew I had only started to scratch the surface. I wished I could sit down individually with each of them, and I cursed myself for not even having prepared a hand-out to give them.

The last person to leave was a woman in her thirties with a kind face and soft grey eyes. I recognized her – she had been in the audience the day before. 'I just had to come back,' she explained. 'I have learnt more from you in one day than I learnt from all the guys with the PhDs – I used to sit through boring seminars while I was training to be a nurse and couldn't wait to leave. But what you are saying makes perfect sense.' This woman later came to my classes, and like many she writes to me regularly to let me know how she is progressing. She always signs herself 'Your No. 1 Fan'.

I was completely exhausted after these three days and was looking forward to a few days' rest before starting my classes again. Ger took me out for dinner that night to celebrate.

'What next then, Bernie?' he asked. 'Today, the RDS Dublin – tomorrow, what? How are you going to top this?'

'I don't know. I was asked if I'd do the show next year – with a bigger room, and I said I'd do the show, but I wasn't sure about the bigger room.'

'Oh, go for it. Anyway, you've plenty of time to think about it.'

'OK. But I'll need to have a proper leaflet to give people. I wonder if I need an e-mail address or a website? People kept asking me if they could contact me.'

'I'd just keep it simple for now if I were you.'

We were to find out 'what next' the following day. I had a call from the TV station Ireland AM. She had heard about my talks at 'Your Health' and wanted me to appear the following week on the breakfast show to talk about what she called my 'system for beating cancer'. Television! This was starting to get serious – I felt panicky. A million questions rushed through my mind. What time? What will I wear? Will I bring anything with me?

'Are you selling or promoting anything?' she asked.

I was aghast. 'Of course not!'

'In that case we can pay you 64 euros.'

I laughed to myself. Not only was I getting an opportunity to appear on television but I was getting paid as well – be it ever so small. She was apologetic, but explained that the people they usually had on their programme tended to be promoting a product or a service, so their telephone numbers and e-mail address or website would be flashed up on the screen at the end of the slot. 'Well, you don't need to do that for me as I have nothing to sell – I just want to tell people how to make these simple changes. I guess I'm not your regular kind of guest.' We agreed on a date, and she told me where the studio was, and what time to arrive.

'Ger!' I yelled, as I put the phone down. 'Help!'

If I had been nervous for the health show I was out of my mind with terror now. I questioned everyone I knew for any tips they might have on how to behave, where to look (The presenter? The cameras? The basket of fruit, my only prop?), what colours to wear … the only thing I wasn't worried about was what to say.

In the reception room next door to the TV studio just before I was due to go on air I asked one of the researchers what I was to expect. 'Oh, the presenter will ask you a few questions. Just act natural. OK, the news is just finishing. You're on now – follow me.' Clearly I was light relief in between news flashes. Off I went, best foot forward.

The presenter that morning asked me, off-camera, if I would talk about chemotherapy. This was a no-no for me. 'I am not qualified to talk about medical treatments, just my own experience,' I said. 'Please, don't even go there. This is a subject I never give advice on, because I feel strongly that each individual should make this decision for themselves. All I want to do is show people the few simple changes I made in my life.'

Suddenly he was all smiles. This was it. I took a deep breath and hoped my nervousness would not show. 'And I'm delighted to introduce Bernadette Bohan,' he announced to the cameras, 'health advisor and cancer survivor.' I was not sure about the label of health advisor, but I launched into my prepared sound bites. 'Juicing is an easy way to get five to ten raw fruit and veg a day,' I began, and the thought crossed my mind that I could do this thing blindfold; I had said these words so many times. I concentrated on making it sound fresh and exciting. It was all over very quickly, and I was ushered out to make way for the next guest. As I left, the studio asked if I could give them some answers for some e-mails and calls they had just received. E-mails and calls? I thought. I've only just come off the air.

On my way home I wondered if any of my friends had seen me, and how I had come across.

'Mum!' cried Sarah as soon as I got home. 'The phone is hopping!' I was bewildered. What had happened?

'What do you mean?' I asked.

'Can I take your number? We'll call you back,' Sarah was saying. Then she held the phone off the hook to talk to me.

'It's you! All these people want to speak to you. As soon as you came off the TV the phone started going. I think they called the TV station and they gave them our number.' She put the phone down and it rang immediately.

'Hello, yes that's right. Can I take your number? Bernadette will call you back.'

I sat down heavily on the sofa, hardly comprehending what was happening. I had no idea of the power of a five-minute television slot. Did this happen to everyone? Why hadn't they warned me? I was glad now that I had an e-mail address – my friend Veronica had set up the account the day before and in the event the TV station had put my e-mail details up on the screen after my slot. I hadn't allowed them to do the same with my phone number – on Ger's advice – but they'd still given it to viewers who had called in. This was just as well, as it turned out, as I was able to help so many.

'I'll man the phone, Sarah. Can you run up and check the e-mails for me?'

'Sure. You were great, by the way.'

For the next two hours I was on the phone non-stop to people who had seen the breakfast show and wanted to know more. Some of them were sick, and all of them wanted to talk. I had to be strong and not get into involved conversations, promising caller after caller that I'd take their number and call them back. Sarah reappeared.

'E-mails are arriving every few minutes,' she reported. 'There are loads of them already. What shall I do with them?' I put my head in my hands.

'Look, let's have a break,' I said. 'I need to feed Julie – the poor little lass has just been pottering around quietly while all this has been going on. I think she needs a bit of normality.' I took the phone off the hook and we had tea. I was worried about the e-mails: it was all very well having an e-mail address, but I didn't know one end of a computer from the other and I couldn't type. How was I going to reply to them all? In the end we decided that Sarah would print them, I would scribble replies on the hard copies, and she would type them up and send them off. I was relieved at this solution and agreed to pay her a few bob for helping me out – I knew it would take her some time to get through all of them.

After Julie was in bed I tentatively put the phone back down, and immediately it rang. The answerphone seemed to be jammed. I lost count of the number of calls I fielded, but I was there for hours. I stopped for a while when Ger came home, and I could see he was both pleased and a bit put out that I was so preoccupied.

'It will quieten down tomorrow, I expect,' he said confidently.

It didn't. The next day I was on the phone for seven hours, and wrote around fifty e-mails for Sarah to send. That night we debated whether to install a new, dedicated phone line, and decided not to, at least for the time being. For three nights Sarah was up until 2am working on the hundreds of e-mails – she was amazing, and I could see how touched she was by some of the stories that were coming through. We had to take the phone off the hook in order to sleep, eat and talk. Richard helped me with Julie so I could be free to take the calls. There were times when I had to remind myself that I had to look after myself: I needed to rest, I needed to eat properly. We had been totally unprepared for this and it was overwhelming. People were asking for more – an information pack, a video, a book, water filters, juicers, sprouting kits. 'I'm not a business,' I kept protesting. 'I'm just telling people how I made myself well after cancer.'

The researcher was on the line again. 'We have had a massive response,' she said excitedly, and admitted that they had been completely taken aback by the amount of calls. 'You certainly captured their interest. We'd like you to come back and do six more slots.'

I knew I wanted to do this. This was a great opportunity, and it was the best way of reaching more people. Next time I would set myself up so as to be able to respond better to queries. We decided I would do one slot every three weeks for the next few months, which would take me up until the following April.

Meanwhile my classes continued, and I found I was booking people in for months ahead. However, there were so many new people that I had to re-jig my waiting lists and see the sick people first: I couldn't possibly make someone with cancer wait two months – it was imperative that they discovered what they could do to help themselves immediately. I had to pace myself to cope with the increased demand, and sadly I was no longer able to see people one-to-one. Letters were still flooding in, and it was so heartening for me to have these daily reminders that people felt

I had genuinely helped them. I was getting stories of tumours regressing, scans being clear, bloods improving (a clear indicator of health). One of these was Susie Halpin. She was suffering from ovarian cancer that had spread to her lung, and after two full treatments of chemotherapy had been told by her oncologists that there was no guarantee that she would not need more treatment. Her daughter saw me on television and contacted me on her mother's behalf, after which her husband John travelled a hundred miles to take my classes and find out what he could do to support her. She wrote recently to tell me that they were headlong into my health plan:

'John has lost 2 stone: he is like a new man and says you are a breath of fresh air. I'm doing very well at the moment, my bloods are excellent and the doctors are very pleased with me. Thank God I'm happy again, and thank you for watching out for me, and for being there for me when I was frightened.'

Over the years I have become close to many people like Susie, corresponding with them, talking with them on the phone, living through the stages of their illnesses with them. I feel blessed to have made so many new friends. It embarrasses me to be given presents, and to be called an 'angel', but I understand their very human need for reassurance and information. Not all survive, it is true; but if they have gained extra time from following my advice then I feel I have done a little for them. I give out a lot of myself, I realize, but I get it back one thousand fold.

I still see my oncologist, and at my last appointment he didn't ask me how I was, he asked me what I was up to. I laughed. I had told him only a little about the changes I had made to my life: with his traditional medical views he would, I feared, pour scorn on what I was doing. I knew full well that he regarded me as one of his success stories. It amused me to think that he had heard about my television appearances and was unsettled by what I was advising people to do. 'When this book comes out I will say that I believe it was the chemo that saved you,' he declared, a little pompously. 'I never said it wasn't,' I replied, smiling. One day I may tell him that doctors now recommend my classes to their patients.

My family is now more accepting of the lifestyle I have chosen, and although I allow them a small weekly ration of three pizzas, one packet of biscuits and one carton of orange juice (I wear dark glasses to buy them!), they do at least have some understanding of the principles I am following. Julie has taken the rollercoaster of the past few years in her stride, and her teacher recently told me that she is now more than able to keep up with the rest of the class. I'm so proud of her.

My brother-in-law, Tony, is a librarian, and he had been on at me for a couple of years to write a book about my experiences. 'I wouldn't know where to start!' I would always protest. But then more and more people were asking me if I was going to write a book, and I realized that this was the logical next step. It would also be wonderful to have something tangible to give out to people, although I couldn't for the life of me imagine how I might do it. Eventually I sent a few pages to a publisher.

To my surprise they accepted it, and here it is: my life in paper-back. It has had its sad moments, but thankfully it has a happy ending.

When people go through a life-threatening illness there are various stages they go through. I see this all the time in the people who come to my classes. Not everyone is the same, of course, but there is often shock and anger at first, followed by denial, but eventually comes acceptance, and a sense of peace and healing – of the mind if not also of the body. This is sometimes referred to as a 'journey', and although I'm wary of labels like this it does seem strangely like a journey to me. As I write these words I am about to turn fifty, and it seems a good moment to reflect on those milestones that brought me here.

My journey has taken me beyond healing to a place where I am able to help others to help themselves, and that in turn adds to my own sense of purpose. I have also noticed that things seem to happen at the right time – is this pure coincidence, or is some greater Power at work? My illness led to my desire for informa-tion; my acquisition of information helped restore me to health and inspired me to tell others. My classes and lectures led to my talk at the big health show, which in turn led to the television slots. The publicity led to the writing of this book with my new friend Jane Ross-Macdonald. The experience of working on the book has brought so many things back to me that I feel I can empathize even more with the people who are now contacting me for help. Everything has fallen into place. And now, I hope, I am contributing to the bank of information from which people can draw their own sustenance on their own journeys – whether they are sick like I was, or whether they are enjoying good health and want to stay that way. I don't know where my journey will take me next, but I thank you for accompanying me through my story this far.

But please don't stop here. In the next few pages I have laid out, as simply as I can, the basics of my health plan. I call it 'Change Simply'.

It is the most important part of the book.

Chapter Nineteen

Change Simply

'When in the grips of disease it is seldom that one renders the courage and commitment to change their circumstance. Bernadette is a living example of what is possible when you honour and respect your life. Be well.'

BRIAN R. CLEMENT,
DIRECTOR, HIPPOCRATES HEALTH INSTITUTE

'Bernadette is a woman whose courage and care are born of the dramas of personal suffering. Health is much simpler than we've been led to believe; in a world where experts make health appear too complex to understand, Bernadette shows that health can be simple and practical.'

UDO ERASMUS, PHD
NUTRITIONIST AND AUTHOR

This section is designed to be an easy-to-follow guide for you to start making the changes to your lifestyle that I guarantee will make you feel better. It is a short version of what I teach people in my classes, and I have laid it out in a step-by-step format so that you can incorporate the easiest changes first.

This is where you will learn why people have been beating a path to my door. There are four sections: juicing, water, foods and safe personal care. I explain my recommendations, and how to go about them. In order to help you get started, I have listed some useful information, including names and addresses of suppliers, at the end of the book. Obviously this is not exhaustive so do check the internet too.

Remember, I am just an ordinary woman. This 'health plan' is the result of extended research on my part and from talking to all the experts I could find. Anything that didn't add up, anything that was recommended in one place and advised against in another – I re-checked again and again, and took what made sense to me. You will see that this plan draws heavily on what is available from Mother Nature, with an emphasis on enzymes. These are the catalysts which break up and assimilate food, and because they are so important you will read repeatedly about them here. I want you to think about what you are putting into your shopping trolley, what you are putting into your mouth and which toiletries and other products you are exposing your body to.

I believe that these simple changes not only helped to save my life, but improved it beyond measure. Are they expensive? Well, you'll need to invest in a juicer and a new water system, and you'll start putting different foods in your shopping trolley. But what I have found, with myself and with the people I have taught, is that as you become more aware of eating better, you naturally stop buying expensive, convenience junk food.

Don't immediately reject these suggestions: remember I do call it change *simply*. I believe that if I, a mother of three demanding kids and on chemo, can make these changes in my life then so can you. Through my classes and lectures I have seen many hundreds of people already change over with not much difficulty. If you are fit and healthy, then you may decide to try one or two of the steps. If you are facing a health problem, then you urgently need to make some changes to your lifestyle now.

The choice is yours. Is it worth it? I think so.

Change a little. It helps a lot.

Step One: Juicing

Why Juice?

Because it is raw and full of enzymes. For me, this was a wonderful first change to make: it is easy and delicious, and I immediately felt the benefits. Juicing is a tasty way of increasing your intake of live vitamins, enzymes and minerals – and all without any artificial colourings, flavours or preservatives. It is the healthiest step you can take for your body, and here's why:

• Recommended Daily Amounts

We already know, thanks to the media, that we ought to be consuming at least five portions of fruit and vegetables per day. Evidence suggests now that the figure should be closer to ten pieces. Juicing enables you to consume these greater quantities (and if you have children, juicing is a great way of getting more raw veggies into them). The point of increasing our intake is to provide our bodies with enough vitamins, minerals, enzymes and trace elements that it needs to fight disease and stay healthy. Processed foods are empty foods.

- A New Trend (actually, the oldest trend)

What we should know, but often overlook, is that eating these foods *raw* is far, far better than eating them cooked, for heating them above 43°C destroys almost all the enzymes (the most important group), nearly all the vitamins and some of the minerals. Even steaming is not as healthy as you might think: the high temperatures required to cook them means that, again, you are destroying the nutrients. With juicing, everything is *raw*, and raw fruits and vegetables retain the nutrients needed by the body for good health. Digesting food is one of the hardest jobs your body has to do, but when it is in juice form, rather than as whole fruits or vegetables, we can digest and assimilate their precious nutrients much more easily. Indeed, they are of particular value to people fighting disease, people with digestive problems or low energy levels. Although juicing eliminates some fibre which is important to health, in the course of the day this can easily be taken through food.

- Time

In just two 250ml glasses of juice per day you can consume around ten portions – ten separate pieces of fruit and vegetables that you would otherwise spend the entire day attempting to chew your way through. It takes about five minutes to make a juice and five minutes to clean up after. They should be consumed within fifteen minutes of preparation, while the enzymes and nutrients are at their best. If you are going out and decide to take a juice with you, store it in a stainless-steel vacuum flask with ice to slow down oxidation of the juice.

- Weight

If you have a weight problem, you will know that all diets allow you to eat as many vegetables as you like, although you should go easy on fruit as many fruits have a high sugar content and will lead to increased weight. Watermelon is a good fruit to use in juice as it has a low sugar content. Juices will fill you up between meals and reduce food cravings.

- Hydration

Juicing enables you to up your fluid intake, which is essential for a healthy body and good skin. (See Step Two on Water for more on hydration.)

- Taste

For me, this is one of the most obvious advantages. So much tastier than any packaged juices or cordials, when I try out my favourite juices on my friends and students they can't wait to get started.

Getting Started

There are two types of juicer on the market – this is an area where there is much confusion as to the best juicer to buy. Having done quite a bit of research before purchasing a masticating juicer, and having survived with a centrifugal juicer for some time, the following analysis of their relative effectiveness is not just my own opinion – it has been echoed by many experts I have spoken to.

Centrifugal juicers are cheaper and readily available in the high street, but I don't recommend these as they:

- can be wasteful (too much pulp produced)
- extract mostly the water from the fruit and veg (clearly seen in the separation of the juice)
- can destroy nutrients due to the heat produced from fast-moving blades
- are difficult to clean (quite off-putting when you are just starting!)

Masticating juicers are used in natural health-care clinics throughout the world. They are more expensive, but certainly worth it. I favour them because they grind, crush and press the fruit and vegetables slowly rather than cut and shred (the speed is 110 revs per minute rather than 3000 revs per minute from the centrifugal type). The advantages of masticating juicers are that they:

- produce good quality juice full of nutrients and enzymes

- produce little pulp, and the pulp that is produced can be passed through the machine again and again to squeeze more juice from it
- are simple to clean
- are excellent for juicing leafy green vegetables and wheatgrass

What Now?

One large glass of fresh juice a day is a good start. Buy more fruit and vegetables when you go shopping, and gradually you will get a feel for how much you will be needing on a weekly basis. When you are ready to start, you can try the following powerful combinations. You will notice I do not give individual amounts as I think this only complicates what is a very simple process. Use whatever you have available:

- Grape and Apple: tasty and sweet, a very popular juice. Always use apple seeds as they contain nitrilosides which protects us from disease (see p. 266 for more on this). Grapes contain selenium and zinc, and are good sources of antioxidants.
- Apple and Carrot: hugely appealing to children, both in taste and colour. Carrots are rich in calcium, phosphorus, potassium, folic acid and carotenoids like beta-carotene. It is particularly good for the eyes and bones.
- Celery and Cucumber; Parsley and Spinach: a combination of two or more of these juices is excellent for clearing up digestive problems, constipation and bad breath. I often think we are obsessed with cleaning our bodies on the outside and ignore the importance of cleaning the inside. Green juices are

superb cleansing juices, and taken first thing in the morning they can move mountains (if you get my meaning).

— Celery is high in potassium, a good source of Vitamin C and loaded with enzymes.

— Cucumbers are mostly water, but they contain numerous enzymes, beta-carotene (which the body converts to Vitamin A), Vitamin C, calcium, phosphorus, iron and potassium. They are often used to remove harmful substances (such as uric acid) from the bloodstream.

— Parsley is high in iron, which helps anaemic conditions. It can also inhibit tumour-cell growth.

— Spinach is rich in L-glutathione, beta-carotene, folic acid, Vitamin C, iron and magnesium. It also contains potent antioxidants and plenty of fibre.

• Wheatgrass: this is the fastest-selling health food on the planet, and has become very popular because of its therapeutic value. Known as a 'superfood', it is extremely effective at fighting disease. It contains high quantities of minerals and is one of the richest sources of beta-carotene, and Vitamins C and B17, a substance that is said to destroy cancer cells. Indeed, it is so powerful that 1 oz of wheatgrass is said to be equivalent to over 2 lb of fresh fruit and vegetables in terms of vitamins, minerals, trace elements and phytonutrients. Today it is sold in many juice bars, but you can also try growing and juicing your own. It can be grown very easily from seed on a windowsill – the whole process takes about ten days. When first juicing wheatgrass you might find the flavour improved by combining the juice with lemon or celery juice.

The above suggestions are just a few ideas to get you started. I hope you enjoy the different tastes, let alone the benefits that juicing will bring to you. Remember: keep it simple, and enjoy it.

Step Two: A Clean Choice

'Few things are as insidious as bad water. It's dangerous for you and your children, but you usually can't tell if you have it. And if you do, you may not be able to tell where the problems are coming from.'

NATIONAL GEOGRAPHIC MAGAZINE,
SPECIAL WATER EDITION, NOVEMBER 1993

Why?

It should not be news to any of us that we need to drink more water – after all, our bodies are made up of about 70 percent water. Water, crucially, is the agent which flushes out toxins, aids digestion and prevents premature ageing and disease in the cells of our bodies. Sufficient water keeps us healthy, cleanses our system internally and gives our skin a gorgeous healthy glow. It's importance cannot be stressed too highly.

Lack of sufficient water, on the other hand, can cause the following:

- premature ageing: sagging of skin, breakdown in cell structure

- a huge variety of illnesses, from asthma and ulcers to high blood pressure and arthritis
- a general feeling of lethargy, headaches and tiredness
- constipation

We can be dehydrated without realizing it – thirst is actually the *last* sign of our body's craving for water, so in fact we should be drinking even when we don't feel thirsty. Don't fool yourself that because you drink plenty of liquid in the form of coffee and tea, sugary or fizzy drinks you are hydrated: these are all diuretics which actually cause your body to *lose* water, and caffeine leeches essential nutrients from the body.

There has been an explosion in the past few years of the sales of bottled mineral water, but:

- Plastic bottles contain oestrogens which can pass into the water.
- Spring and mineral waters contain dissolved solids which are difficult for the body to digest. (The body's need for minerals is met through foods: plants pick up minerals and make them available to us.)
- Quite apart from anything else, bottled water is expensive.

What about tap water? I know many people who feel bottled water is a rip-off and insist on a large jug of tap water when they are eating out – but what exactly is in our water supply? I'm afraid the news is not good, and just because the water coming out of your tap looks clear and fresh does not mean that it is clean. Think before you drink.

Tap water contains certain dangerous substances that are added to the drinking supply:

- *Fluoride* is not approved for human consumption in any country in the world, and has never been safety-tested on humans. It damages bones and enamel, it is not recommended in pregnancy, and is unsuitable for babies. Fluoride accumulates in the skeleton, joints and glands and is linked to irritable bowel syndrome, cancer, arthritis and osteoporosis. According to Dr Dean Burk, the chief chemist from the US National Cancer Institute, fluoride causes more human cancer deaths than any other chemical. It has been rejected or banned by Austria, Belgium, Denmark, Finland, France, Germany, Holland, Italy, Northern Ireland, Norway, Portugal, Scotland, Sweden, Switzerland, Wales and most of England. More insidiously, new studies have pointed to a link between fluoride and chromosomal damage. It has been used as rat-poison. Fluoride is a by-product of aluminium mining and contains high concentrations of heavy metals such as lead and arsenic – proven carcinogens. Surely here are just about enough reasons not to want this in our water, don't you think?

But what about teeth, you will ask? Preventing tooth decay by adding fluoride to our water makes little sense as it creates an unacceptable toxic health hazard. All the evidence I have seen suggests that the jury is still out on fluoride being of any real benefit to our teeth. A recent Report for the Department of Health and Social Security in the UK stated that 'no essential function exists for fluoride in the diet'. The truth is that cavities are caused by bacteria and excessive acidity, not lack of fluoride, and good dental hygiene is the answer. Many health stores now stock safe alternatives (more of this in Step Four: Safe Personal Care).

- *Chlorine* was used during World War I to gas people. Now it is added to our water supply because it is a cheap disinfectant which kills harmful bacteria (although not – it is important to note – the nasty bugs E. coli and Cryptosporidia). This is a good idea in principle, but unfortunately this practice may be hazardous to human health. While it destroys harmful bacteria, chlorine also kills good bacteria in the digestive system, it destroys Vitamin E, and can form chloroform, a known carcinogen. Studies have shown links with increased risk of heart disease, as well as many cancers, including prostate, colon, bladder and rectal. Chlorinated water also has an unpleasant taste and smell. Perhaps this is why we are all so dehydrated?
- *Aluminium* is used to clarify the water. It also potentiates the effects of heavy metals like mercury, lead and cadmium – which are all present in our drinking water. The links of aluminium's toxic effects with Alzheimer's are well documented.

OK, so I think you have got the picture by now. The tap water we drink is not safe, despite modern treatment stations, and despite the best efforts of the water authorities. Quite simply, it is too expensive to clean our water sufficiently to make it healthy to drink. Indeed, even if today's water-treatment facilities were able to purify water completely, it would become re-contaminated by old, leaky and outdated water mains and pipes.

It follows that what we need is natural, pure water. Water that does not 'take' or 'give' nutrition. Water that simply does the job it is intended to do: hydrate all the cells of our bodies so they can work efficiently.

We need to clean up the water coming into our homes. It is an easy and effective step to take, and I'll tell you how.

How to Clean Your Water

Plastic jugs with water filters are limited in their effectiveness. These merely use a screen to separate only particles of dirt sediment from water. The good news is that there are two very effective water systems currently available:

- Distilled Water

The use of a home distiller is a very effective way of cleaning your water and leaving it free of contaminants. Tap water is heated to 100° centigrade, a temperature at which bacteria, germs, viruses and cysts are killed. The steam rises, leaving behind dissolved solids, chemicals, salts, contaminants and impurities. This steam then condenses into distilled water – water just about as clean as you can get. These distillers are available in portable, compact units (at the lower price range) or larger more permanent units (higher priced). The smaller units need quite a bit of cleaning so they are not always suitable for busy families.

- Reverse Osmosis

This filtration system uses the principle of reverse osmosis to remove 95–98 per cent of all the mineral and chemical contaminants from raw tap water. Reverse osmosis was originally designed to make sea water drinkable for the Navy. You may remember from your schooldays how osmosis works: if a salt solution and a water solution are separated by a membrane, the water will pass through the membrane to reach the salt in order to achieve equilibrium. It is the process by which our cells absorb nutrients. Using this system, by reversing the process the two are separated again – salt and contaminants on one side; pure water on the other. Reverse osmosis uses a semi-permeable membrane that removes not only particles but a very high percentage of dissolved contaminant molecules from water. Several separate filters remove rust, dirt, chlorine, organic chemicals, multi-chemical compounds and micro-organisms and bacteria. The system usually fits under your sink unit and has a separate tap that you can have installed on your kitchen work-surface or sink, and gives you an unlimited supply of good drinking water. It is easy to maintain, and the filters only need to be changed once a year.

Getting Started

Both these systems give you water which is clean, fresh and delicious, and I'm sure it will encourage you to drink it in preference to fizzy drinks, coffees and teas. It takes time to adjust to drinking larger amounts of water, and gradually you will get used to it. Adding some lemon juice and warming it to body temperature is a very easy way to consume those extra few glasses that your body so desperately needs. As an added benefit, your kettle will no longer fur up with lime deposits. Thanks to the purity of the water produced, both these systems are used within medical and pharmaceutical laboratories, which I think is a pretty good recommendation. Check the Resources section at the end of this book for ideas on where to find a system to suit you. They are not cheap, but in the long run much safer, more convenient and economical than buying gallons of bottled water.

Your body will immediately feel the benefits.

Step Three: Powerful Foods

In my experience most people find that any changes to the food they eat are the most challenging to make. I have found it best to find alternatives and add them to the diet before eliminating those foods you are already used to.

In this section I will tell you about some powerful food groups which you can add to your diet to make your body stronger at fighting disease. I want you to feel positive about the changes, because only then will you actually incorporate them into your lifestyle.

The good news is that to put good foods back into our diet is easy.

Nitrilosides

One group of foods you should know about are the Vitamin B17 foods, or nitrilosides. They have been called the 'missing link' in our modern diet. Before the Industrial Revolution our bread was made with millet, a rich source of B17. Around the beginning of the last century it was discovered that wheat was easy to grow and cheaper to produce, and this one massive agricultural change took that important source of B17 away from the population. In countries where people consume foods rich in B17, there are lower rates of degenerative diseases such as heart disease, cancer and arthritis. Studies show that nitrilosides are highly effective in protecting us from disease. Fortunately, Nature has provided us with many common foods which contain these nitrilosides.

Wheatgrass is the richest source, but humans can only digest this in juice. Other good sources include apricot kernels, apple seeds, pear seeds, bitter almonds, walnuts, pecans, blackberries, gooseberries, cranberries, buckwheat, lentils and millet. And – wait for it – sprouts!

Sprouts

The greatest boon to my diet – in terms of what I eat, rather than drink – has without question been the discovery of sprouting. These little seedlings contain so much of the vital health-giving nutrients that they simply cannot be ignored. Foods that are sprouted contain the most concentrated and easily assimilated forms of the nutrients we are in desperate need of. They are one of the best natural sources of vitamins, minerals, enzymes and amino acids (which are proteins in a digestible form). I include sprouts I have grown in my own kitchen in sandwiches, salads, stews, cereals, juices and soups. They are always fresh, they are cheap to produce, and – although you can find them in some organic supermarkets – anyone can grow them. They can also be slipped unobtrusively into family meals!

Sprouting is a wonderful source of nutrition that can be prepared in your own kitchen, and takes about five minutes a day. From three to four ounces of seeds you can produce five litres of sprouts. When activated by moisture and warmth, a huge amount of life force is released: they begin to grow, and after a few hours they begin to release Vitamin C, a process which continues for up to a week. After a few days they release the B vitamins. They also contain protein, vitamins A, B-complex, C, D and E, enzymes, iron, potassium, magnesium, calcium, amino acids and essential fatty acids.

Sprouts have been found to:
- protect against cancer, arthritis, heart disease and other illnesses
- help the body to flush out waste
- improve immune system function
- improve mood and vitality

Getting Started

You will need a few clean wide-necked glass jars covered with net or muslin secured with an elastic band; and a selection of organic seeds – available from health-food stores (not garden centres!).

1. Soak the seeds in their jars in water overnight or for 6–12 hours.
2. Rinse and drain. They should be placed at a 45-degree angle so the water drains off.
3. Rinse and drain the sprouts twice daily.
4. When the sprouts have grown, place in indirect sunlight.
5. After a day or two small green leaves will appear.
6. They are now ready to eat. Put a lid on the jar and refrigerate.
7. They can be stored for up to a week. (If they have not sprouted, or you forget to rinse them, throw them out and start again.)

Some of the easiest seeds to start with, to my mind, are the following:

Alfalfa
Red clover
Fenugreek
Onion
Sunflower
Sesame
Pumpkin

Some Powerful Supplements

This is an area I would like to touch on as I believe many people spend a lot of money on supplements and are often confused as to what to buy. So here are the basics, as I call them. I am often asked my opinion on supplements, and my advice is to obtain nutrients through food. I don't advise people to take supplements because I have found the scientific evidence too contradictory, and if you are juicing you will be getting high doses of nutrients direct from Mother Nature. However, I do make an exception for these three supplements – essential fats, enzymes and probiotics.

Essential Fats

These are also known as omega-3 and omega-6 fats. They are not produced by the body, so we must supply the body and the brain with these fats. Because of recent trends towards low-fat diets, most of us are so low in these essential nutrients that our bodies cannot survive properly without them. Before I list a few of the benefits (too many to describe here!), let me first say this as clearly as I can:

Essential fats do not make you fat.
Excessive carbohydrates make you fat.

If you restrict your carbohydrate intake you will not gain weight. It is essential to feed the brain – it is a large organ and must be supplied with essential fatty acids. Some of the most common signs of deficiency of these fats are dry skin conditions such as eczema, as well as acne, allergies, water retention, and a sluggish metabolism – which can result in obesity.

The benefits

Essential fats are nature's moisturizers, making skin soft and velvety smooth and forming a barrier against loss of moisture and dehydration. Dry skin is not life-threatening, so the body will rob from the skin to supply the vital inner organs. You can obtain excellent results with essential fatty acids against eczema, acne and psoriasis; you will tan better and burn less. Essential fats increase metabolic rate and noticeably boost energy levels which increases calorie burning. These fats keep us slim! Essential fats also balance hormones and reduce the symptoms of PMT and the menopause, which is good news for women. They greatly assist in reducing inflammation and improving mobility in the joints where arthritis is a problem, thereby reducing pain and discomfort. They significantly help children suffering from dyslexia, hyperactivity and attention deficiency.

Sources

Essential fats are easy to obtain in seed oils such as flax, sunflower and sesame. They are also present in oily fish but as most fish harbour parasites and sometimes environmental poisons, healthy fats from fish might be accompanied by some less desirable substances. Seeds oils should be refrigerated or they will become completely ineffective. You can add these oils to food (your body will absorb them more easily) such as salad dressings, mashed potato, or steamed vegetables. Start with small amounts, gradually increasing to allow your body to adjust. Your skin and hair will love these fats.

Enzymes

I have mentioned enzymes in the sections on juicing and sprouting, and here they are again. Enzymes are behind every chemical and muscle action in your body, from digestion to the repair of damaged tissue. They convert the foods we eat into smaller, usable nutrients and play a key role in all the body's systems.

Enzymes come from two sources: internal and external. Internally, the digestive system secretes enzymes in saliva, gastric juices, and in the pancreas and intestine. External enzymes are best found in raw food. Nature endows all raw food with the enzymes required for its digestion. Modern food-processing techniques and cooking methods destroy almost 100 per cent of these enzymes needed for the vital job of breaking down and absorbing food. Our diets no longer contain as much raw food as they once did. Our bodies also produce fewer digestive enzymes as we age or if we are ill. Cooked food, alcohol, stress and micronutrient deficiencies also take their toll on our enzymes reserves and decrease production. This combination puts enormous strain on our digestive system.

Food allergies, gas, bloating, digestive upsets, weakened immunity, low energy levels – these can all be signs of insufficient enzymes. If we can take on more live, enzyme-rich foods in the form of juices, sprouts and raw food it saves the body from using up its own enzymes, freeing it up to concentrate on staying healthy. Enzymes protect our cells from free-radical damage, and as such they help protect us against the ageing process. Wow! Enzymes are at the heart of my Change Simply plan.

An enzyme supplement is one of the most powerful supplements available. Everyone can benefit from using digestive enzymes to improve digestion and nutrient absorption. People with digestive problems can obtain excellent results in a relatively short time. These are what I discovered when I was unable to keep food down during my chemotherapy treatment and the benefit was immediate. They can be taken in capsule form, or the capsule can be opened and sprinkled on cold or warm (but not hot) food. This is not a supplement to ignore.

Probiotics

Poor eating habits and the use of antibiotics in food production, as well as medical treatments, can wreak havoc on the delicate balance of our gastro-intestinal tract and immune system. Probiotic supplements can be of benefit for a wide variety of conditions. They enhance the immune system and prevent unfriendly organisms from gaining a foothold in the body. They are amazing at preventing overgrowths of yeasts and fungal infections. They are recommended for candida, for instance, because they establish large healthy populations of friendly bacteria that compete with candida, and can be used externally to combat a variety of yeasts and fungal infections. Probiotic capsules can be broken open and the contents placed in socks or underwear, and they can also be taken orally. Probiotics also provide protection against mouth ulcers and sore throats, and can impair the growth and activity of the harmful bacteria that are responsible for intestinal disorders such as E. coli and salmonella. They are highly recommended during and after courses of antibiotic treatment. Friendly bacteria also protect against the harmful effects of radiation and pollutants.

One important fact to remember when buying probiotics – refrigeration ensures maximum potency and stability, and they can only be left un-refrigerated for short periods of time. They work best if taken immediately after meals when the acidity of the gastric juices has been diluted by food and is not as concentrated.

Probiotics are absolutely essential for proper digestion, strong immune function and overall health. They are a must for your home remedy kit.

*

I have chosen the foods and supplements in this section because of the powerful effects they can have on our bodies. Don't underestimate the value of food: it keeps us alive.

Step Four: Safe Personal Care

The cosmetic industry spends billions of dollars each year persuading us that we need their products. We assume these products are safe, yet there are many harmful chemicals used in day-to-day products like toothpaste, shampoo, deodorant, moisturizers, body lotions and make-up. Our generation is the first to be exposed to the dangers of these harmful chemicals, and not only are we exposed to these products, we are persuaded to buy them by some of the most sophisticated advertising techniques of our day. So check your labels, just as you do with food, and beware of words such as 'natural', 'organic' and 'hypoallergenic' – these merely mask the truth behind these prettily packaged toiletries, cosmetics and soaps.

1. *Fluoride:* I have talked about the dangers of fluoride in our water, and this same danger exists in toothpaste. America's labelling laws are many years ahead and more stringent than ours, and on toothpaste packaged in the US a sign now appears by law: 'If more than is needed for brushing is accidentally swallowed, contact a poisons control centre immediately.' As little as 1g ingested can cause dangerous poisoning. Fluoride accumulates in body tissue and can be poisonous when ingested over long periods of time. We use this dangerous substance twice or three times a day. Surely something that is this toxic shouldn't be going into our mouths.

2. *Sodium Lauryl Sulphate* is a harsh detergent used in commercial shampoos and toothpaste. When ingested it is more toxic than if it were taken intravenously. It is rapidly absorbed and readily penetrates the skin. It is also retained in the eyes, brain and liver – particularly in the eyes of the young, and its effect in the liver and brain is cumulative. Skin allergies, contact eczema and cataracts (and mouth ulcers, in the case of toothpaste) are some of the risks we are exposing ourselves to when we use this harsh chemical. It has been found to cause liver and skin cancer in animal studies – and yet it is used in many children's shampoos and bubble bath. There are many safe shampoos on the market. Make the change.

3. *Aluminium* found in antiperspirants is highly toxic to humans. The removal of this chemical from antiperspirants has been called for by the FDA (Food and Drug Administration) advisory panel in the United States. A positive link with Alzheimer's disease has been proven by recent research which found the brains of victims contained large amounts of aluminium. Breast cancer, DNA damage and osteoporosis are other dangers associated with this chemical, and products containing aluminium compounds are listed as suspected carcinogens. The continuous use of antiperspirants containing these suspected carcinogens makes no sense to me when there are so many safe alternatives readily available.

4. *Propylene Glycol:* this is a strong skin irritant that is systemic, and can get into the bloodstream. It is found in many skin-care products, make-up, body lotion, baby wipes and hair products because it prevents the escape of moisture. It is also found in paint, liquid laundry detergents, anti-freeze and brake fluid. Safety data sheets are supplied when this product is used in industry stipulating that the user must avoid skin contact. It weakens the immune system and has been found to cause kidney damage and liver abnormalities. Do you still feel comfortable using this on your skin or wiping your baby with this chemical?

So what do you do about all this scary stuff? Simple. Just buy products from health shops, on-line, or from distributors (see Resources section) that are safe. There are many alternatives, and once you know what to look out for, it's easy. Remember these four:

- Fluoride and sodium lauryl sulphate in toothpaste
- Sodium lauryl sulphate and sodium laureth sulphate in shampoos
- Aluminium in antiperspirants
- Propylene glycol in skin and hair-care products

AND FINALLY ...

Three Essential Cancer-Fighting Tips

I have read so many health books that I know how easy it is to miss out on the small truths, which often turn out to be the most vital information the book holds. So I have decided to keep until last these three essential tools for fighting cancer.

Each one of us has cancers growing inside us from time to time. What stops them growing and getting out of hand is a healthy immune system, so it is imperative that we keep ours in healthy working order.

1. *Drink*
   We cannot survive without water. Drink as much as you can: two to three litres a day is crucial for cellular hydration. Flush out the toxins and give your body this pure life-giving elixir. And make sure it's clean.
2. *Sugar*
   Cancer feeds on all forms of sugar. Refined sugar has been connected to a host of diseases: diabetes, cancer, arthritis, heart disease, Crohn's disease and obesity. I know it's hard to take,

but we must find cancer's Achilles heel. Like the rest of us, cancer loves this sweet poison.

3. *Exercise*

   Cancer hates oxygen. In 1931 a chemist named Otto Warburg discovered that a lack of oxygen causes cancer. He was given the Nobel Prize for this discovery. His conclusion was that oxygenating the cancer cell was the best way to fight cancer as well as viruses, bacteria and fungal infections. It follows that exercise, which oxygenates the body, will help ward off disease. So get moving.

Well, there you have it: in a nutshell, the foundations of the health plan that changed my life. Fresh juice, clean water, a few key foods and safe personal-care products. I have sifted through a lot of information in order to try to make this section of the book as short and to the point as possible, and I truly hope that it will inspire you to make these simple changes in your own life.

I wish you good health.

Resources

Recommended Products, Companies and Organizations

Green Star Masticating Juicers and Water Distillers

Naturalife Health Ltd
Rathnew
Ireland Tel: 0404 62444
info@naturalife.ie
www.naturalife.ie

Savant Distribution Ltd
Quarry House
Clayton Wood Close
Leeds
LS16 6QE
UK
Tel: 08450 60 60 70
info@savant-health.com
www.savant-health.com

Reverse Osmosis Systems

Reverse Osmosis Ltd
Dundalk
Co Louth
Tel: 087 2473173
business@reverseosmosis.ie
www.reverseosmosis.ie

Udo's Choice Oil Blend, Udo's Digestive Enzymes Super 8 & 5, plus Speciality Supplements and organic seeds for sprouting

Naturalife Health Ltd
Rathnew
Ireland
Tel: 0404 62444
info@naturalife.ie
www.naturalife.ie

Savant Distribution Ltd
Quarry House
Clayton Wood Close
Leeds LS16 6QE
UK
Tel: 08450 60 60 70
info@savant-health.com
www.savant-health.com

Flora Inc. (distributors of Udo's products)
PO Box 73
805E Badger Road
Lynden
Washington
USA 98264
Tel: 18004462110
www.floralhealth.com

Safe Personal-Care Products

Available from good health-food stores, plus:

Forever Natural UK
The Old Barrel Store
Brewery Courtyard
Drayman's Lane
Marlow, Bucks
SL7 2FF. UK
Tel: 01628 891700
Fax: 01628 891701

The Natural Medicine Company
Burgage
Blessington
Co Wicklow
Ireland
Tel: 045 865575

Neways International
Tel: 042 9377328
philip@renewell.com

Neways United Kingdom
Tel: 01480 861764
info@neways.co.uk
www.neways.co.uk

Organic Food Delivery Services

An Talamh
Tel: 0596 473460
marylstap@eircom.net

Organic Delights
Tel: 087 2485826
organicdenishealy@hotmail.com

Healing Centre

Hippocrates Health Institute
1443 Palmdale Court
West Palm Beach
Florida 33411
USA
Tel: 561 471 8876
www.hippocrates.inst.com

Useful Websites

www.voice.buz.org
www.irishlivingfood.com
www.cancerdecisions.com

To contact Bernadette Bohan:
b@changesimply.com
www.changesimply.com

Recommended Reading

General

Brian Clements, *Living Foods for Optimum Health*, Prima Health, 1998

Phillip Day, *Cancer: why we're still dying to know the truth*, Credence Publications, 1999

Phillip Day, *Food for Thought*, Credence Publications, 2001

Siegfried Gursche, *Encyclopaedia of Natural Healing*, Alive Books, 1997

Jane Plant, *Your Life in Your Hands*, Virgin Books, 2000

Steven Ransom, *Great News on Cancer in the 21st Century*, Credence Publications, 2002

Andrew Weil, *Spontaneous Healing*, Little, Brown, 1995

Chris Woollams, *Everything You Need to Know to Help You Beat Cancer*, Health Issues Ltd, 2002

Juicing

Siegfried Gursche, *Juicing – for the health of it*, Alive Books, 2000

Jason Vale, *The Juice Master's Ultimate Fast Food*, ThorsonsElement, 2003

Caroline Wheater, *Juicing for Health*, Thorsons, 2001

Water

Tonita d'Raye, *What's the Big Deal About Water?* The Ten Minute Read Company, 1995

Lono Kahuna Kupua A'O, *Don't Drink the Water*, Kali Press, 1996

Foods

Udo Erasmus, *Fats that Heal, Fats that Kill*, Alive Books, 1993

Lynne Melcombe, *Health Hazards of White Sugar*, Alive Books, 2000

Kathleen O'Bannon, *Sprouts*, Alive Books, 2000

Safe Personal Care

Dr Stephen & Gina Antczak, *Cosmetics Unmasked*, Thorsons, 2001

David Steinman & Samuel S. Epstein, *The Shoppers' Bible*, Wiley
Publishing Inc., 1995

P.M. Taubert, *Silent Killers – more than you paid for*, CompSafe
Consultancy, 2001

excellent book - powerfull -
Simply change - it works
and Bio energy Re aligns
heals and helps.
definitely works* Noirin Fogarty *
Life coach, Bio energy + Cranial -
Sacral therapist (gentle healer)
@; noirin.fogarty@gmail.com Dublin
Tel; 086 - 3870321.
This is not me - but a friend angel
and highly qualified healing lady,
" what she does, works."
Caroline Woods 085-108579